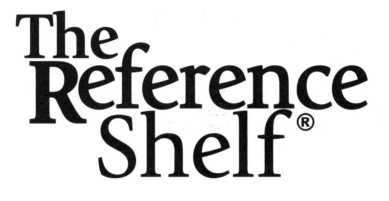

The
Reference
Shelf®

Global Epidemics

Edited by Christopher Mari

The Reference Shelf
Volume 79 • Number 2

The H. W. Wilson Company
2007

The Reference Shelf

The books in this series contain reprints of articles, excerpts from books, addresses on current issues, and studies of social trends in the United States and other countries. There are six separately bound numbers in each volume, all of which are usually published in the same calendar year. Numbers one through five are each devoted to a single subject, providing background information and discussion from various points of view and concluding with a subject index and comprehensive bibliography that lists books, pamphlets, and abstracts of additional articles on the subject. The final number of each volume is a collection of recent speeches, and it contains a cumulative speaker index. Books in the series may be purchased individually or on subscription.

Library of Congress has cataloged this serial title as follows:

Global epidemics / edited by Christopher Mari.
  p. ; cm.—(Reference shelf ; v. 79, no. 2)
 Includes bibliographical references and index.
 ISBN 978-0-8242-1068-7 (alk. paper)
 1. Epidemics—History. 2. Avian influenza. 3. Bioterrorism. I. Mari, Christopher. II. Series.
 [DNLM: 1. Disease Outbreaks—history—Collected Works. 2. Disease Outbreaks—prevention & control—Collected Works. 3. Bioterrorism—psychology—Collected Works. 4. Orthomyxoviridae Infections—prevention & control—Collected Works. 5. World Health—Collected Works. WA 105 G5625 2007]
  RA649.G56 2007
  614.4—dc22

                   2007001533

Cover: Photo By Justin Sullivan/Getty Images

Visit H. W. Wilson's Web site: www.hwwilson.com

Printed in the United States of America

Contents

Preface

By presenting articles on a wide variety of subjects and from a broad range of authors, this volume will provide a general understanding of the history of epidemic outbreaks and the means by which we as a civilization can combat them collectively. As the World Health Organization, the United Nations, and various national institutes of medicine have noted, it is only through international efforts that epidemic outbreaks can be contained and lives saved.

The term "epidemic," which is derived from the Greek *epi*, meaning "upon," and *demos*, meaning "people," is defined here as an outbreak of infectious disease that spreads through a human population at a faster rate than what has been recorded in recent incidences. Though "epidemic" is often used metaphorically to discuss a host of societal issues, from the spread of illegal drug use to the cell-phone craze, this volume will focus exclusively on the *medical* definition of the term. Endemic disease, or maladies that occur at steady if debilitating rates in certain areas, such as malaria in tropical climates, will not be discussed to any great degree. Because it would be impossible to cover *every* epidemic that has occurred throughout history in a volume of this size, several infamous and illustrative examples, both historic and current, will be highlighted in order to give the reader a sense of an outbreak's magnitude and power.

Epidemics have existed throughout recorded human history. Though defining what constitutes an actual outbreak has proven somewhat subjective, the impact of an epidemic on humanity has not: AIDS, smallpox, the Black Death, and other diseases have exacted incalculable tolls from mankind, threatening entire societies and destroying ways of life. While poorer countries and regions tend to be more susceptible to epidemics, no nation, no matter how wealthy, is invulnerable. Though it may initially be contained in a certain locale, such as a city or town, an epidemic has the potential to develop into a larger outbreak impacting not only nations, but entire continents, and indeed the whole world. When a disease spreads across the planet, it is known as a pandemic. One of the more notable examples of such a phenomenon in recent history is the Great Influenza Pandemic of 1918–19, also known as the "Spanish Flu," which first emerged in the trenches of World War I before spreading across the globe. Within 12 months it killed at least 50 million people—and did so in an era before modern transportation could disseminate the disease more effectively. Consequently, if such an outbreak were to occur today, in an age when people (and the germs they carry) can travel across the planet in a matter of hours, the toll could be even greater. Given the common interest in forestalling such an eventuality, crafting an effective international response, one that emphasizes both prevention and containment, is of vital concern to the global medical community.

This book is divided into five sections, the first of which, "Notable Epidemics in Human History," features articles discussing the origin and evolution of the term "epidemic" and exploring several of the more historically devastating outbreaks, among them the bubonic plague, smallpox, cholera, the Spanish Flu, polio, and AIDS. Pieces in the second section, "Preventing, Controlling, and Eradicating Epidemic Outbreaks," examine the various methods employed to combat epidemics in a globalized world and offer critiques of current strategies to contain the spread of such contagions as AIDS and tuberculosis. "Is Avian Flu the Next Epidemic?" the book's third chapter, includes entries analyzing whether or not the "bird flu," which has spread from poultry to humans in recent years, will emerge as the next pandemic and, if so, whether the international medical community is up to the task of containing and counteracting it. Setting the medical challenges aside, the fourth chapter, "The Psychological and Economic Impact of Epidemics," presents articles debating the potential impact a widespread outbreak would have on the global economy and community. Pieces in the final section, "Bioterrorism," discuss the threat posed by terrorists seeking to use biological agents to spark an epidemic outbreak and whether such fears are warranted.

In closing, I would like to thank Joseph Miller and Lynn Messina for the opportunity to edit this book, as well as Richard Stein and Paul McCaffrey for their invaluable contributions to its production. A special thank you goes to my wife, Ana Maria Estela, whose love, support, insight, and knowledge helped guide this volume from its conception to its final form.

Christopher Mari
April 2007

I. Notable Epidemics in Human History

Editor's Introduction

As stated in the Preface, epidemic disease has always been part of the human experience. While a variety of conditions may exacerbate the toll of a particular epidemic—war, commerce, or poor sanitation, for example—and the means of transmission may vary considerably—be it via insect bite, bodily fluids, or airborne pathogens—the one commonality that binds all epidemics together is the degree to which they are social phenomena. Indeed, it is humanity's interconnectedness, our ties to one another, that makes epidemics so deadly. Nevertheless, we have remained social creatures, believing that the value of our collective endeavors outweighs the security that an antiseptic isolation might provide.

The first section of the book serves as an introduction to the topic of global epidemics, broadly defining the term and presenting several infamous historical examples of deadly pathogens to demonstrate how these diseases were transmitted and what the infected communities did to combat them. In the first article, "The 2,500-year Evolution of the Term Epidemic," Paul M. V. Martin and Estelle Martin-Granel chart the evolving meaning of the word "epidemic." Noting how the term first appears in the works of the ancient poet Homer and entered the medical lexicon when Hippocrates used it as the title of one of his well-known treatises in 430 B.C., the authors demonstrate how the meaning of the word has changed over the years, taking on its current definition during the Middle Ages.

In "The Black Death: The Greatest Catastrophe Ever," Ole J. Benedictow recounts the horrors of the bubonic plague, contending that the disease, which spread across Europe between 1346 and 1353, killed more people than had been previously estimated. Benedictow believes 50 million people, or roughly 60 percent of what was then the continent's total population, succumbed to the malady.

Mark Thomson considers the devastating impact of smallpox on the Native American population after it was introduced to the New World following Christopher Columbus's arrival in 1492 in the third entry, "The Migration of Smallpox and Its Indelible Footprint on Latin American History." In "Sick City," Steven Shapin recalls how a physician named John Snow used scientific observations to trace the cholera epidemic plaguing London in 1848 to a contaminated water supply.

Next, Nell Boyce, in "Flu's Worst Season," describes how scientists are working with recovered genes from the Spanish Flu to explain why that particular strain of influenza exacted such a devastating toll in 1918 and 1919. Renee Skelton, in "Conquering Polio," details the various polio epidemics that crippled or killed many Americans, as well as how this destructive disease was ultimately cured. The final article in this section, "How AIDS Changed America," by David Jefferson, chronicles the evolution of the American understanding of this deadly virus over the last 25 years.

2,500-year Evolution of the Term Epidemic

BY PAUL M. V. MARTIN* AND ESTELLE MARTIN-GRANEL†
EMERGING INFECTIOUS DISEASES, JUNE 2006

The term epidemic (from the Greek epi [on] plus demos [people]), first used by Homer, took its medical meaning when Hippocrates used it as the title of one of his famous treatises. At that time, epidemic was the name given to a collection of clinical syndromes, such as coughs or diarrheas, occurring and propagating in a given period at a given location. Over centuries, the form and meaning of the term have changed. Successive epidemics of plague in the Middle Ages contributed to the definition of an epidemic as the propagation of a single, well-defined disease. The meaning of the term continued to evolve in the 19th-century era of microbiology. Its most recent semantic evolution dates from the last quarter of the 20th century, and this evolution is likely to continue in the future.

At the start of the 21st century, epidemics of infectious diseases continue to be a threat to humanity. Severe acute respiratory syndrome, avian influenza, and HIV/AIDS have, in recent years, supported the reality of this threat. Civil wars and natural catastrophes are sometimes followed by epidemics. Climate change, tourism, the concentration of populations in refugee camps, the emergence of new human pathogens, and ecologic changes, which often accompany economic development, contribute to the emergence of infectious diseases and epidemics[1]. Epidemics, however, have occurred throughout human history and have influenced that history. The term epidemic is ≈ 2,500 years old, but where does it come from?

Before Hippocrates

When works that put forward new ideas are translated, determining the original terminology (in Ancient Greek in this case) is not easy. In 430 BC, when Hippocrates was collecting the clinical observations he would publish in Epidemics, his treatise that forms the foundation of modern medicine, at least 3 terms were used in Ancient Greece to describe situations that resembled those described by Hippocrates: *nosos*, *phtoros*, and *loimos*[2].

* Institut Pasteur de Nouvelle Calédonie, Nouméa, New Caledonia; and

† Collège Enseignement Secondaire Le Bosquet, Bagnols-sur-Cèze, France

Article by Paul M. V. Martin and Estelle Martin-Granel from *Emerging Infectious Diseases* June 2006. Copyright © *Emerging Infectious Diseases*. Reprinted with permission.

Nosos, meaning disease, was used by Plato in the 4th century BC and clearly had the same meaning 2 centuries earlier in the works of Homer and Aeschylus. Nosos encompasses disease of the mind, body, and soul: physical, including epilepsy, and moral (i.e., psychological and psychiatric). Phtoros or *phthoros* means ruin, destruction, deterioration, damage, unhappiness, and loss, after war for example. The word was frequently used by Aeschylus and Aristophanes, was known in the 8th century BC, and was later used by Plato and Thucydides. Its meaning has remained general. Bailly translates loimos as plague or contagious scourge. Used by Esiodus in the 7th century BC and later by Sophocles and Herodotus, this term is ancient. Its translation as plague should be interpreted in the sense of a scourge rather than as the disease plague. In the Septuagint, a translation of the Old Testament into Greek by 70 Greek Jews from Alexandria, this word is used in the book of Kings to describe the 10 plagues of Egypt.

But the term epidemic already existed in 430 BC. The Greek word *epidemios* is constructed by combining the preposition *epi* (on) with the noun *demos* (people), but demos originally meant "the country" (inhabited by its people) before taking the connotation "the people" in classical Greek. Indeed, the word epidemios was used by Homer, 2 centuries before Hippocrates, in the Odyssey (canto I, verses 194 and 230), where it was used to mean "who is back home" and "who is in his country" in contrast to a voyager who is not :δὴ γάρ μιν ἔφανι 'ἐπιδήμιον εἶναι σὸν πατέρα,"because someone said that your father was back (home)" (canto I, verse 194). In this context, epidemios means indigenous or endemic. In the Iliad, Homer confirmed this meaning (canto XXIV, verse 262), by using also *polemos epidemios* to mean civil war: "this one who ὃς πολέμου ἔραται ἐπιδημίου οκρυόευτος liked passionately the frightening civil war" (canto IX, verse 64). Later, Plato and Xenophon (400 BC) used the word to describe a stay in a country or the arrival of a person:Παριος ὄυ ἐγὼ ἠσθόμην ἐπιδημοῦντα, "a Parian who, I learned, was in town" (Plato, Apology, chapter I, paragraph 38). The verb *epidemeo* was used by Thucydides (460 BC–395 BC) to mean "to stay in one's own country," in contrast to *apodemeo*, "to be absent from one's country, to travel." For Plato, epidemeo meant "to return home after a voyage, to be in town." Later, the orators Demosthenes (384 BC–322 BC) and Eschines (390 BC–314 BC) used this word to refer to a stranger who came to a town with the intention of living there, and the verb epidemeo was used to mean "to reside." Typical of Greek semantics, epidemeo takes its meaning from the result of the action, rather than from the action itself. It relates to something that has already happened, with the implication that it had previously happened elsewhere. Authors before Hippocrates used epidemios for almost everything (persons, rain, rumors, war), except diseases. Hippocrates was the first to adapt this word as a medical term.

Hippocrates and the Term Epidemic

Written in the 5th century BC, Hippocrates' Corpus Hippocraticum contains 7 books, titled Epidemics[3]. Hippocrates used the adjective epidemios (on the people) to mean "which circulates or propagates in a country"[4]. This adjective gave rise to the noun in Greek, *epidemia*.

We do not know why Hippocrates chose epidemios to title his books instead of nosos, a well-established term meaning disease. Examining the meaning of the term before, during, and after his time may help us understand his choice. Schematically speaking, epidemios (or epidemeo) was used successively to mean "being at homeland" (Homer), "arriving in a country" or "going back to homeland" (Plato), and later "stranger coming in a city" (Demosthenes). Sophocles (495 BC–406 BC) used the adjective in Oedipus Tyrannos to refer to something (a rumor, noise, fame, or reputation) spreading in a country: εἶμ' Οἰδιπόδα ἐπὶ τ'αν ἐπίδαμον φ'ατιν, "I shall go (to make war) to Oedipus, against his fame which spread (in the country)" (verse 494). Oedipus Tyrannos was written at approximately the same time as Corpus Hippocraticum; consequently, we can infer that during Hippocrates' time, epidemios acquired a dynamic meaning, probably more adapted to describing a group of physical syndromes that circulate and propagate seasonally in a human population (i.e., on the people) than nosos, a term used to describe diseases at the individual level.

How epidemios, meaning "on the people," became adapted to mean "that which circulates or propagates in a country" is a crucial question. This evolution occurred during the second half of the 5th century (450 BC–400 BC), a period of intense activity in Greek literature, particularly with the prolificacy of Sophocles. But while nosos or loimos were frequently used, epidemios was not. In the Perseus Digital Library (www.perseus.tufts.edu), a database that does not yet include Hippocrates' works, the adjective epidemios was used only 9 times, including 4 times in Homer, in the 489 major referenced Greek texts ($\approx$4.8 millions words, 0.02 occurrences per 10,000 words). Its Doric variants *epidamos* and *epidemos* were used 3 times. In comparison, nosos (disease) was used 712 times in the Perseus database (1.47 occurrences per 10,000 words). The verb epidemeo was used 144 times, primarily during the 4th century and always meaning "to live in or return to one's own country." This lack of material makes accurately exploring the reasons for the semantic evolution across centuries difficult. In Oedipus Tyrannos, Sophocles qualified the sense of epidemios as it referred to reputation or fame; fame naturally spreads in a country. But Hippocrates described a series of syndromes: καὶγαρ ἄλλως το νούσημα ἐπίδημον ἦν, "It is a fact that the disease was propagating in the country" (Epidemics, book 1, chapter 3). Although Sophocles used epidemios once in that new sense, Hippocrates established a medical meaning for the term.

In Epidemics, books I and III constitute lists of diseases describing clinical cases. Hippocrates compared these cases and grouped them to generate series of similar cases. He adopted a classification approach, initially seeking clinical similarities between cases, thereby discovering, in addition to the notion of epidemic, the more fundamental concepts of symptom and syndrome. However, Hippocrates believed that prognosis was a major aspect of medicine. This belief led him to consider disease a dynamic process with its own progression, a temporal dimension, that represents a first nosologic evolution: syndromic groupings become diseases. Another of the books written by the physician from Kos—Airs, Waters, and Places—deals with the relationships between diseases and the environment, focusing particularly on the habitat of the patients and the season in which disease occurs. Hippocrates tried to determine the effect of environmental factors on what could be described as the distribution of diseases. He was, thus, more concerned about group-

---

Hippocrates tried to determine the effect of environmental factors on what could be described as the distribution of diseases.

---

ing together winter diseases or autumn diseases or diseases that occurred in a particular place or in persons whose way of life had changed than in identifying a large number of cases of the same disease in winter or autumn, at a particular place, or in association with a particular way of life. For Hippocrates, whose nosologic approach already contained a major element of preoccupation with the environment, the first meaning of epidemic was groups of cases resembling each other clinically and the second meaning was groups of different diseases occurring at the same place or in the same season and sometimes spreading "on the people." Thus, Hippocrates applied the word epidemios to groupings of syndromes or diseases, with reference to atmospheric characteristics, seasons or geography, and sometimes propagation of a given syndrome in the human population.

Semantic confusion caused the great Emile Littré, who translated Hippocrates' works into French in the first half of the 19th century, to make a nosologic error. Hippocrates described what is known today, since the work of Littré, as the Cough of Perinthus. This account can be found in Epidemics book VI. Hippocrates described coughs that started toward the winter solstice and were accompanied by many symptoms: sore throat, leg paralysis, peripneumonia, problems with night vision, voice problems, difficulty swallowing, difficulty breathing, and aches. When Littré published his translation and commentaries on Epidemics in 1846, he mistakenly considered the Cough of Perinthus to be a single disease[5]. This error made retrospectively diagnosing the diseases of Perinthus difficult, if not impossible. Moreover, as Littré saw this collection of illnesses as a single disease, he essentially turned it into an epidemic, probably because he had the modem sense of the term in mind and thought that Hippocrates had observed and described an epidemic illness unknown to modern medicine[5].

According to Grmek, "Littré took chapter VI, 7.1 as a general description of an epidemic in the sense of this word in the medical language of the 19th century rather than in the sense intrinsic to the works of Hippocrates. In the Corpus Hippocraticum, the noun 'epidemic' designates a collection of diseases observed at a given place, during a given period. A disease described as epidemic, such as epidemic cough, is a condition occurring from time to time in a given place, the appearance of which is closely linked to changes in season and climatic variations from year to year"[5].

Historians of medicine and philologists have over the years attributed the Cough of Perinthus to diphtheria, influenza, epidemic encephalitis, dengue fever, acute poliomyelitis, and many other diseases. However, a French physician named Chamseru, who practiced in the 18th century, almost a century before Littré, finally got to the bottom of what may be meant by the Cough of Perinthus, probably because the term epidemic had not yet taken on the meaning it had in Littré's time. According to Chamseru, the Cough of Perinthus could have encompassed several diseases, among them diphtheria, influenza, and whooping cough[5].

Thucydides and the First Descriptions of Epidemics

Thucydides (460 BC–395 BC) interrupted his account of the Peloponnesian War to describe the famous Plague of Athens, which occurred at the start of the summer in 430 BC. This description was long considered among the first descriptions of an epidemic. Indeed, whereas Thucydides used nosos, the term plague, which is used by all the translators of his work, is used in the sense of the Latin term *pestis*, a term with no clear etymology[4], meaning contagious disease, epidemic, or scourge. The description of the Plague of Athens, like that of the Cough of Perinthus by Hippocrates, is an essential text in the philologic and semantic study of epidemics[5]. We must therefore consider, as for Littré's translation, the meaning that translators have assigned to the original description by Thucydides. Thucydides never used the term epidemic that Hippocrates was in the process of establishing. Under the term nosos, Thucydides described a series of clinical signs, which originated in the south of Ethiopia and propagated throughout Egypt, Libya, and then Greece. Thucydides used the words nosos, *kakos* (evil), *ponos* (pain), phtoros (ruin, destruction), and loimos (scourge) to describe what his translators call plagues. In her translation of Thucydides' works[6], published in 1991, in the chapter titled Second Invasion of Attica: the Plague of Athens (the original Greek work had no title), Jacqueline de Romilly translated nosos as disease or epidemic. Similarly, she translated loimos, kakos, and phtoros as disease or epidemic and the list of clinical signs (the original Greek meant "following these things") as symptoms. de Romilly rendered the text more elegant and accessible to 20th-century readers by this translation but gave the words used by Thucydides their 20th-century meaning rather than the meanings they had in the 5th century BC. Herein lies the principal problem of translation.

But was the Plague of Athens a true epidemic, in the modern sense? The death rate for the disease was extremely high, reaching up to 25% in 1 group of soldiers, and Pericles died of it. Historians have tried to understand the origin of this plague, and various diseases have been suggested, e.g., typhus, measles, smallpox, bubonic plague, ergotism, or an unknown disease. Thucydides wrote that all preexisting diseases were transformed into a plague and that persons in good health were affected in the absence of a predisposing cause[7]. The large number of symptoms and of possible and probable

---

This evolution [of the term epidemic] is representative of the evolution of science and medicine over the centuries and reflects the semantic evolution of the term.

---

causes rules out the possibility of an epidemic in the modern sense of the term. Instead, the Plague of Athens seems to have been the appearance of a large number of diseases that affected the population at the same time. Plague therefore has the same meaning here as epidemic in the works of Hippocrates. These 2 terms have been used in association or confused throughout history. However, epidemic existed at this time, even if the notion of epidemic as we mean it in modern times had not yet emerged.

Evolution of the Term Epidemic

After the nonmedical use of the term epidemic by Homer, Sophocles, Plato, and Xenophon, Hippocrates gave it its medical meaning. However, the term has since undergone a long evolution. The adjective epidemios gave rise to the Greek noun *epidemia*. The Greek term epidemia in turn gave rise to the Latin term *epidimia* or *epidemia*. The term *ypidime* in Medieval French has its origins in these Latin words and went on to become *épydime* in the 14th century, *epidimie* in the 17th century, and then *epidémie* in the 18th century. Not until 22 centuries after Hippocrates, in the second half of the 19th century, were the terms *épidémiologie* (1855), *épidémiologique* (1878), and *épidémiologiste* (1896) coined in French and notions attached to them developed. Of course, at approximately the same time, corresponding terms appeared in the English language. The term epidemic and the terms linked to it therefore required an extremely long time to be constructed. This evolution is representative of the evolution of science and medicine over the centuries and reflects the semantic evolution of the term.

Semantic Evolution

In parallel with the evolution of the term epidemic itself, its meaning also changed over time. If we limit ourselves to the meaning that epidemic has acquired with respect to infectious diseases, we can identify 4 major steps in its semantic evolution in the medical sense. For Hippocrates, an epidemic meant a collection of syndromes occurring at a given place over a given period, e.g., winter coughs on the island of Kos or summer diarrheas on other islands. Much later, in the Middle Ages, the long and dramatic succession of waves of The Plague enabled physicians of the time to identify this disease with increasing precision and certainty; they began to recognize epidemics of the same, well-characterized disease. Then, with the historic contributions of Louis Pasteur and Robert Koch, epidemics of a characteristic disease could be attributed to the same microbe, which belonged to a given genus and species. The last stage in the semantic evolution of the term epidemic was the pro-

TABLE: SEMANTIC EVOLUTION OF THE TERM EPIDEMIC		
STAGE IN EVOLUTION	MEANING	USE
Greek: EPI (on) and DEMOS (people) (6th century BC); EPIDEMIOS used by Homer in the Odyssey	Who is in his country	Nonmedical use
Greek: Sophocles and Hippocrates (second half of the 5th century BC)	That which circulates and propagates in a country	First medical use
Greek: EPIDEMIOS established by Hippocrates (430 BC) in the medical sense of a collection of syndromes	Sometimes spreading "on the people"	Epidemic of diarrhea
Medieval French: EPIDIME (1256 and late, EPIDIMIE)	Large number of cases of unique, well-characterized disease	Epidemic of cholera
19th century: ÉPIDÉMIE (late 18th-century French) and EPIDEMIC (18th-century English)	Epidemics caused by a microbe belonging to a given genus and species	Epidemic of cholera due to VIBRIO CHOLERAE
End of 20th century	Clonal expansion of an epidemic strain, as defined with molecular markers	An epidemic due to V. CHOLERAE El Tor, belonging to a defined ribotype or pulsotype

gressive acquisition of the notion that most epidemics were due to the expansion of a clone or clonal complex of bacteria or viruses known as the epidemic strain[8]. More recently, microevolution of a clone of a bacterium (the epidemic strain) was shown to occur during an epidemic with person-to-person transmission[9]. The Table summarizes these 4 major stages in the semantic evolution of the term epidemic.

In the second half of the 20th century, epidemic was also applied to noninfectious diseases, as in cancer epidemic or epidemic of obesity. The extension of the meaning to noninfectious causes refers to a disease that affects a large number of people, with a recent and substantial increase in the number of cases. This semantic extension of epidemic also concerns nonmedical events; the term is used by journalists to qualify anything that adversely affects a large number of persons or objects and propagates like a disease, such as crack cocaine or computer viruses.

What can we gain from investigating the origin and meaning of the word epidemic or from studying its semantic evolution? Beyond simply satisfying our curiosity, the slow evolution of the form and meaning of the term suggests that we still have much to learn about the concept of epidemic.

Acknowledgments

We thank Jean-Michel Alonso and Jean-Pierre Dedet for thorough reading and criticism of the manuscript.

Dr Martin is a bacteriologist and *chef de laboratoire* at the Pasteur Institute and director of the Pasteur Institute of New Caledonia. His research interests focus on epidemics.

Ms Martin-Granel is a *professeur certifiée de lettres classiques* and teaches French literature, Latin, and Ancient Greek in secondary school in the south of France. She has recently translated a text by Petrarch into French.

References

1. Morse SS. Factors in the emergence of infectious diseases. Emerg Infect Dis. 1995;1:7–14.

2. Bailly A, Dictionnaire grec–français. Paris: Payot; 1950.

3. Littré E. Oeuvres complètes d'Hippocrate. Volume II. Paris: Baillère; 1840. p. 598.

4. Rey A. Dictionnaire historique de la langue française. Paris: Dictionnaires Le Robert, 1992.

5. Grmek MD. Les maladies á l'aube de la civilisation occidentale. Paris: Payot; 1994.

6. de Romilly J. Thucydide, la guerre du Péloponnèse, livre II, texte établi et traduit par Jacqueline de Romilly. Paris: Les Belles Lettres; 1991.

7. Carmichael AG. Plague of Athens. In: Kiple KF, editor. The Cambridge world history of human disease. Cambridge: Cambridge University Press; 1993.

8. Wachsmuth K. Molecular epidemiology of bacterial infections: examples of methodology and of investigations of outbreaks. Rev Infect Dis. 1986;8:682–92.

9. Kriz P, Giogini D, Musilek M, Larribe M, Taha MK. Microevolution through DNA exchange among strains of *Neisseria meningitidis* isolated during an outbreak in the Czech Republic. Res Microbiol. 1999;150:273–80.

The Black Death

The Greatest Catastrophe Ever

By OLE J. BENEDICTOW
HISTORY TODAY, MARCH 2005

The disastrous mortal disease known as the Black Death spread across Europe in the years 1346–53. The frightening name, however, only came several centuries after its visitation (and was probably a mistranslation of the Latin word "*atra*" meaning both "terrible" and "black"). Chronicles and letters from the time describe the terror wrought by the illness. In Florence, the great Renaissance poet Petrarch was sure that they would not be believed: "O happy posterity, who will not experience such abysmal woe and will look upon our testimony as a fable." A Florentine chronicler relates that,

> All the citizens did little else except to carry dead bodies to be buried [. . .] At every church they dug deep pits down to the water-table; and thus those who were poor who died during the night were bundled up quickly and thrown into the pit. In the morning when a large number of bodies were found in the pit, they took some earth and shovelled it down on top of them; and later others were placed on top of them and then another layer of earth, just as one makes lasagne with layers of pasta and cheese.

The accounts are remarkably similar. The chronicler Agnolo di Tura "the Fat" relates from his Tuscan home town that

> . . . in many places in Siena great pits were dug and piled deep with the multitude of dead [. . .] And there were also those who were so sparsely covered with earth that the dogs dragged them forth and devoured many bodies throughout the city.

The tragedy was extraordinary. In the course of just a few months, 60 per cent of Florence's population died from the plague, and probably the same proportion in Siena. In addition to the bald statistics, we come across profound personal tragedies: Petrarch lost to the Black Death his beloved Laura to whom he wrote his famous love poems; Di Tura tells us that "I [. . .] buried my five children with my own hands."

The Black Death was an epidemic of bubonic plague, a disease caused by the bacterium *Yersinia pestis* that circulates among wild rodents where they live in great numbers and density. Such an area

---

is called a "plague focus" or a "plague reservoir." Plague among humans arises when rodents in human habitation, normally black rats, become infected. The black rat, also called the "house rat" and the "ship rat," likes to live close to people, the very quality that makes it dangerous (in contrast, the brown or grey rat prefers to keep its distance in sewers and cellars). Normally, it takes ten to fourteen days before plague has killed off most of a contaminated rat colony, making it difficult for great numbers of fleas gathered on the remaining, but soon-dying, rats to find new hosts. After three days of fasting, hungry rat fleas turn on humans. From the bite site, the contagion drains to a lymph node that consequently swells to form a painful bubo, most often in the groin, on the thigh, in an armpit or on the neck. Hence the name bubonic plague. The infection takes three–five days to incubate in people before they fall ill, and another three–five days before, in 80 per cent of the cases, the victims die. Thus, from the introduction of plague contagion among rats in a human community it takes, on average, twenty-three days before the first person dies.

> From the introduction of plague contagion among rats in a human community it takes, on average, twenty-three days before the first person dies.

When, for instance, a stranger called Andrew Hogson died from plague on his arrival in Penrith in 1597, and the next plague case followed twenty-two days later, this corresponded to the first phase of the development of an epidemic of bubonic plague. And Hobson was, of course, not the only fugitive from a plague-stricken town or area arriving in various communities in the region with infective rat fleas in their clothing or luggage. This pattern of spread is called "spread by leaps" or "metastatic spread." Thus, plague soon broke out in other urban and rural centres, from where the disease spread into the villages and townships of the surrounding districts by a similar process of leaps.

In order to become an epidemic the disease must be spread to other rat colonies in the locality and transmitted to inhabitants in the same way. It took some time for people to recognize that a terrible epidemic was breaking out among them and for chroniclers to note this. The timescale varies: in the countryside it took about forty days for realisation to dawn; in most towns with a few thousand inhabitants, six to seven weeks; in the cities with over 10,000 inhabitants, about seven weeks, and in the few metropolises with over 100,000 inhabitants, as much as eight weeks.

Plague bacteria can break out of the buboes and be carried by the blood stream to the lungs and cause a variant of plague that is spread by contaminated droplets from the cough of patients (pneumonic plague). However, contrary to what is sometimes believed, this form is not contracted easily, spreads normally only episodically or incidentally and constitutes therefore normally only a small fraction of plague cases. It now appears clear that human fleas and lice did not contribute to the spread, at least not significantly. The bloodstream of humans is not invaded by plague bacteria from the buboes, or people die with so few bacteria in the blood that blood-sucking human parasites become insufficiently infected to become infective and spread the disease: the blood of plague-infected rats contains 500–1,000 times more bacteria per unit of measurement than the blood of plague-infected humans.

Importantly, plague was spread considerable distances by rat fleas on ships. Infected ship rats would die, but their fleas would often survive and find new rat hosts wherever they landed. Unlike human fleas, rat fleas are adapted to riding with their hosts; they readily also infest clothing of people entering affected houses and ride with them to other houses or localities. This gives plague epidemics a peculiar rhythm and pace of development and a characteristic pattern of dissemination. The fact that plague is transmitted by rat fleas means plague is a disease of the warmer seasons, disappearing during the winter, or at least lose most of their powers of spread. The peculiar seasonal pattern of plague has been observed every-

---

The fact that plague is transmitted by rat fleas means plague is a disease of the warmer seasons, disappearing during the winter.

---

where and is a systematic feature also of the spread of the Black Death. In the plague history of Norway from the Black Death 1348–49 to the last outbreaks in 1654, comprising over thirty waves of plague, there was never a winter epidemic of plague. Plague is very different from airborne contagious diseases, which are spread directly between people by droplets: these thrive in cold weather.

This conspicuous feature constitutes proof that the Black Death and plague in general is an insect-borne disease. Cambridge historian John Hatcher has noted that there is "a remarkable transformation in the seasonal pattern of mortality in England after 1348": whilst before the Black Death the heaviest mortality was in the winter months, in the following century it was heaviest in the period from late July to late September. He points out that this strongly indicates that the "transformation was caused by the virulence of bubonic plague."

Another very characteristic feature of the Black Death and plague epidemics in general, both in the past and in the great outbreaks in the early twentieth century, reflects their basis in rats and rat fleas: much higher proportions of inhabitants contract plague and die from it in the countryside than in urban centres. In the case of English plague history, this feature has been underlined by Oxford historian Paul Slack. When around 90 per cent of the population lived in the countryside, only a disease with this property combined with extreme lethal powers could cause the exceptional mortality of the Black Death and of many later plague epidemics. All diseases spread by cross-infection between humans, on the contrary, gain increasing powers of spread with increasing density of population and cause highest mortality rates in urban centres.

Lastly it could be mentioned that scholars have succeeded in extracting genetic evidence of the causal agent of bubonic plague, the DNA-code of *Yersinia pestis*, from several plague burials in French cemeteries from the period 1348–1590.

It used to be thought that the Black Death originated in China, but new research shows that it began in the spring of 1346 in the steppe region, where a plague reservoir stretches from the north-western shores of the Caspian Sea into southern Russia. People occasionally contract plague there even today. Two contemporary chroniclers identify the estuary of the river Don where it flows into the Sea of Azov as the area of the original outbreak, but this could be mere hearsay, and it is possible that it started elsewhere, perhaps in the area of the estuary of the river Volga on the Caspian Sea. At the time, this area was under the rule of the Mongol khanate of the Golden Horde. Some decades earlier the Mongol khanate

---

The extent of the contagious power of the Black Death has been almost mystifying.

---

had converted to Islam and the presence of Christians, or trade with them, was no longer tolerated. As a result the Silk Road caravan routes between China and Europe were cut off. For the same reason the Black Death did not spread from the east through Russia towards western Europe, but stopped abruptly on the Mongol border with the Russian principalities. As a result, Russia which might have become the Black Death's first European conquest, in fact was its last, and was invaded by the disease not from the east but from the west.

The epidemic in fact began with an attack that the Mongols launched on the Italian merchants' last trading station in the region, Kaffa (today Feodosiya) in the Crimea. In the autumn of 1346, plague broke out among the besiegers and from them penetrated into the town. When spring arrived, the Italians fled on their ships. And the Black Death slipped unnoticed on board and sailed with them.

The extent of the contagious power of the Black Death has been almost mystifying. The central explanation lies within characteristic features of medieval society in a dynamic phase of modernisation heralding the transformation from a medieval to early modern European society. Early industrial market-economic and capitalistic developments had advanced more than is often assumed, especially in northern Italy and Flanders. New, larger types of ship carried great quantities of goods over extensive trade networks that linked Venice and Genoa with Constantinople and the Crimea, Alexandria and Tunis, London and Bruges. In London and Bruges the Italian trading system was linked to the busy shipping lines of the German Hanseatic League in the Nordic countries and the Baltic area, with large broad-bellied ships called cogs. This system for long-distance trade was supplemented by a web of lively short and medium-distance trade that bound together populations all over the Old World.

The strong increase in population in Europe in the High Middle Ages (1050–1300) meant that the prevailing agricultural technology was inadequate for further expansion. To accommodate the growth, forests were cleared and mountain villages settled wherever it was possible for people to eke out a living. People had to opt for a more one-sided husbandry, particularly in animals, to create a surplus that could be traded for staples such as salt and iron, grain or flour. These settlements operated within a busy trading network running from coasts to mountain villages. And with tradesmen and goods, contagious diseases reached even the most remote and isolated hamlets.

In this early phase of modernisation, Europe was also on the way to "the golden age of bacteria," when there was a great increase in epidemic diseases caused by increases in population density and in trade and transport while knowledge of the nature of epidemics, and therefore the ability to organise efficient countermeasures to them, was still minimal. Most people believed plague and mass illness to be a punishment from God for their sins. They responded with religious penitential acts aimed at tempering the Lord's wrath, or with passivity and fatalism: it was a sin to try to avoid God's will.

Much new can be said on the Black Death's patterns of territorial spread. Of particular importance was the sudden appearance of the plague over vast distances, due to its rapid transportation by ship. Ships travelled at an average speed of around 40km a day which today seems quite slow. However, this speed meant that the Black Death easily moved 600km in a fortnight by ship: spreading, in contemporary terms, with astonishing speed and unpredictability. By land, the average spread was much slower: up to 2km per day along the busiest highways or roads and about 0.6km per day along secondary lines of communication.

As already noted, the pace of spread slowed strongly during the winter and stopped completely in mountain areas such as the Alps and the northerly parts of Europe. Yet, the Black Death often rapidly established two or more fronts and conquered countries by advancing from various quarters.

Italian ships from Kaffa arrived in Constantinople in May 1347 with the Black Death on board. The epidemic broke loose in early July. In North Africa and the Middle East, it started around September 1st, having arrived in Alexandria with ship transport from Constantinople. Its spread from Constantinople to European Mediterranean commercial hubs also started in the autumn of 1347. It reached Marseilles by about the second week of September, probably with a ship from the city. Then the Italian merchants appear to have left Constantinople several months later and arrived in their home towns of Genoa and Venice with plague on board, some time in November. On their way home, ships from Genoa also contaminated Florence's seaport city of Pisa. The spread out of Pisa is characterized by a number of metastatic leaps. These great commercial cities also functioned as bridgeheads from where the disease conquered Europe.

In Mediterranean Europe, Marseilles functioned as the first great centre of spread. The relatively rapid advance both northwards up the Rhône valley to Lyons and south-westwards along the coasts towards Spain—in chilly months with relatively little shipping activity—is striking. As early as March 1348, both Lyon's and Spain's Mediterranean coasts were under attack.

En route to Spain, the Black Death also struck out from the city of Narbonne north-westwards along the main road to the commercial centre of Bordeaux on the Atlantic coast, which by the end of March had become a critical new centre of spread. Around April 20th, a ship from Bordeaux must have arrived in La Coruña in northwestern Spain; a couple of weeks later another ship from there let loose the plague in Navarre in northeastern Spain. Thus, two northern plague fronts were opened less than two months after the disease had invaded southern Spain.

Another plague ship sailed from Bordeaux, northwards to Rouen in Normandy where it arrived at the end of April. There, in June, a further plague front moved westwards towards Brittany, south-eastwards towards Paris and northwards in the direction of the Low Countries.

Yet another ship bearing plague left Bordeaux a few weeks later and arrived around May 8th, in the southern English town of Melcombe Regis, part of present-day Weymouth in Dorset: the epidemic broke out shortly before June 24th. The significance of ships in the rapid transmission of contagion is underscored by the fact that at the time the Black Death landed in Weymouth it was still in an early phase in Italy. From Weymouth, the Black Death spread not only inland, but also in new metastatic leaps by ships, which in some cases must have travelled earlier than the recognized outbreaks of the epidemic: Bristol was contaminated in June, as were the coastal towns of the Pale in Ireland; London was contaminated in early August since the epidemic outbreak drew comment at the end of September. Commercial seaport towns like Colchester and Harwich must have been contaminated at about the same time. From these the Black Death spread inland. It is now also clear that the whole of England was conquered in the course of 1349 because, in the late autumn of 1348, ship transport opened a northern front in England for the Black Death, apparently in Grimsby.

The early arrival of the Black Death in England and the rapid spread to its southeastern regions shaped much of the pattern of spread in Northern Europe. The plague must have arrived in Oslo in the autumn of 1348, and must have come with a ship from south-eastern England, which had lively commercial contacts with Norway. The outbreak of the Black Death in Norway took place before the disease had managed to penetrate southern Germany, again illustrating the great importance of transportation by ship and the relative slowness of spread by land. The outbreak in Oslo was soon stopped by the advent of winter weather, but it broke out again in the early spring. Soon it spread out of Oslo along the main roads inland and on both sides of the Oslofjord. Another independent introduction of contagion occurred in early July 1349 in the town of Bergen; it arrived in a ship from England, probably from King's Lynn. The opening of the second plague front was the reason that all Norway could be conquered in the course of 1349. It disappeared completely with the advent of winter, the last victims died at the turn of the year.

> Napoleon did not succeed in conquering Russia. Hitler did not succeed. But the Black Death did.

The early dissemination of the Black Death to Oslo, which prepared the ground for a full outbreak in early spring, had great significance for the pace and pattern of the Black Death's further conquest of Northern Europe. Again ship transport played a crucial role, this time primarily by Hanseatic ships fleeing homewards from their trading station in Oslo with goods acquired during the winter. On their way the seaport of Halmstad close to the Sound was apparently contaminated in early July. This was the starting point for the plague's conquest of Denmark and Sweden, which was followed by several other independent introductions of plague contagion later; by the end of 1350 most of these territories had been ravaged.

However, the voyage homewards to the Hanseatic cities on the Baltic Sea had started significantly earlier. The outbreak of the Black Death in the Prussian town of Elbing (today the Polish town of Elblag) on August 24th, 1349, was a new milestone in the history of the Black Death. A ship that left Oslo at the beginning of June would probably sail through the Sound around June 20th and reach Elbing in the second half of July, in time to unleash an epidemic outbreak around August 24th. Other ships that returned at the end of the shipping season in the autumn from the trading stations in Oslo or Bergen, brought the Black Death to a number of other Hanseatic cities both on the Baltic Sea and the North Sea. The advent of winter stopped the outbreaks initially as had happened elsewhere, but contagion was spread with goods to commercial towns and cities deep into northern Germany. In the spring of 1350, a northern German plague front was formed that spread southwards and met the plague front which in the summer of 1349 had formed in southern Germany with importation of contagion from Austria and Switzerland.

Napoleon did not succeed in conquering Russia. Hitler did not succeed. But the Black Death did. It entered the territory of the city state of Novgorod in the late autumn of 1351 and reached the town of Pskov just before the winter set in and temporarily suppressed the epidemic; thus the full outbreak did not start until the early spring of 1352. In Novgorod itself, the Black Death broke out in mid-August. In 1353, Moscow was ravaged, and the disease also reached the border with the Golden Horde, this time from the west, where it petered out. Poland was invaded by epidemic forces coming both from Elbing and from the northern German plague front and, apparently, from the south by contagion coming across the border from Slovakia via Hungary.

Iceland and Finland are the only regions that, we know with certainty, avoided the Black Death because they had tiny populations with minimal contact abroad. It seems unlikely that any other region was so lucky.

How many people were affected? Knowledge of general mortality is crucial to all discussions of the social and historical impact of the plague. Studies of mortality among ordinary populations are far more useful, therefore, than studies of special social groups, whether monastic communities, parish priests or social elites. Because around 90 per cent of Europe's population lived in the countryside, rural studies of mortality are much more important than urban ones.

Researchers generally used to agree that the Black Death swept away 20–30 per cent of Europe's population. However, up to 1960 there were only a few studies of mortality among ordinary people, so the basis for this assessment was weak. From 1960, a great number of mortality studies from various parts of Europe were published. These have been collated and it is now clear that the earlier estimates of mortality need to be doubled. No suitable sources for the study of mortality have been found in the Muslim countries that were ravaged.

> Researchers generally used to agree that the Black Death swept away 20–30 per cent of Europe's population.

The mortality data available reflects the special nature of medieval registrations of populations. In a couple of cases, the sources are real censuses recording all members of the population, including women and children. However, most of the sources are tax registers and manorial registers recording households in the form of the names of the householders. Some registers aimed at recording all households, also the poor and destitute classes who did not pay taxes or rents, but the majority recorded only householders who paid tax to the town or land rent to the lord of the manor. This means that they overwhelmingly registered the better-off adult men of the population, who for reasons of age, gender and economic status had lower mortality rates in plague epidemics than the general population. According to the extant complete register of all households, the rent or tax-paying classes constituted about half the population both in the towns and in the countryside, the other half were too poor. Registers that yield information on both halves of the populations indicate that mortality among the poor was 5–6 per cent higher. This means that in the majority of cases when registers only record the better-off half of the adult male population, mortality among the adult male population as a whole can be deduced by adding 2.5–3 per cent.

Another fact to consider is that in households where the householder survived, other members often died. For various reasons women and children suffer higher incidence of mortality from plague than adult men. A couple of censuses produced by city states in Tuscany in order to establish the need for grain or salt are still extant. They show that the households were, on average, reduced in the countryside from 4.5 to 4 persons and in urban centres from 4 to 3.5 persons. All medieval sources that permit the study of the size and composition of households among the ordinary population produce similar data, from Italy in southern Europe to England in the west and Norway in northern Europe. This means that the mortality among the registered households as a whole was 11–12.5 per cent higher than among the registered householders.

Detailed study of the mortality data available points to two conspicuous features in relation to the mortality caused by the Black Death: namely the extreme level of mortality caused by the Black Death, and the remarkable similarity or consistency of the level of mortality, from Spain in southern Europe to England in north-western Europe. The data is sufficiently widespread and numerous to make it likely that the Black Death swept away around 60 per cent of Europe's population. It is generally assumed that the size of Europe's population at the time was around 80 million. This implies that that around 50 million people died in the Black Death. This is a truly mind-boggling statistic. It overshadows the horrors of the Second World War, and is twice the number murdered by Stalin's regime in the Soviet Union. As a proportion of the population that lost their lives, the Black Death caused unrivalled mortality.

This dramatic fall in Europe's population became a lasting and characteristic feature of late medieval society, as subsequent plague epidemics swept away all tendencies of population growth. Inevitably it had an enormous impact on European society and greatly affected the dynamics of change and development from the medieval to Early Modern period. A historical turning point, as well as a vast human tragedy, the Black Death of 1346–53 is unparalleled in human history.

For Further Reading

Ole J. Benedictow, *The Black Death, 1346–1353. The Complete History* (Boydell & Brewer, 2004); Ole J. Benedictow, "Plague in the Late Medieval Nordic Countries," *Epidemiological Studies* (1996); M. W. Dols, *The Black Death in the Middle East* (Princeton, 1970); J. Hatcher, *Plague, Population and the English Economy 1348–1530* (Basingstoke, 1977); J. Hatcher "England in the Aftermath of the Black Death" (*Past & Present*, 1994); L. F. Hirst, *The Conquest of Plague* (Oxford, 1953).

The Migration of Smallpox and Its Indelible Footprint on Latin American History

BY MARK THOMSON
THE HISTORY TEACHER, NOVEMBER 1998

When people think of historical migrations, they typically think of human migrations—the Pilgrims or the Mormons, for example. The importance of these migrations is well documented. The importance of disease migration is less obvious, but no less real. One particularly deadly disease, smallpox, visited every continent inhabited by man during its centuries of existence, leaving devastation and misery in its wake. It left something else, too: an indelible footprint on history. As it circled the globe, smallpox killed pharaohs, kings, and emperors. It undermined governments, helped determine the outcome of wars, and shaped the course of exploration and expansion. Nowhere was smallpox's impact more pronounced than in the New World, where it caused the extinction of whole civilizations and dramatically reshaped the cultures of those who survived.

Throughout much of history, word of a smallpox epidemic was the most terrifying news imaginable. This terror was justified; smallpox was a disease "almost unprecedented in its ghastliness."[1] A sixteenth century Franciscan friar described the horrors of a smallpox epidemic among the Indians of present-day Mexico in this way:

> [The smallpox] extended over all parts of their bodies. Over the forehead, head, chest. It was very destructive. Many died of it. They could no longer walk, they could do no more than lie down, stretched out on their beds. They couldn't bestir their bodies, neither to lie face down, nor on their backs, nor to turn from one side to the other. And when they did move, they cried out. In death, many [bodies] were like sticky, compacted, hard grain . . . many [of the survivors] were pockmarked . . . some were blind. . . .[2]

The Historical Origins of Smallpox

No one knows exactly where smallpox originated. Prior to Columbus' discovery of the New World, there is no evidence that smallpox existed in the Americas, although it was, by then, endemic in much of the rest of the world.[3] Smallpox may have originated in northern

Africa, where Egyptian mummies from 1570 to 1055 B.C., including the remains of the Egyptian pharaoh Ramses V, show signs of the disease.[4] References in writings from India suggest that smallpox may also have existed there as early as 1500 B.C.[5] Whatever its origins, smallpox soon spread, probably carried by armies seeking new conquests and merchants engaged in trade. By 430 B.C., smallpox appears to have reached Greece. The Athenian historian Thucydides's description of a mysterious "Plague of Athens," which erupted during the Peleponnesian War, suggests that it was smallpox. According to Thucydides, this epidemic originated in Ethiopia and spread to Egypt and Libya before arriving in Athens on a trade ship.[6] Eventually, smallpox reached Europe. The earliest substantiated evidence of this migration involved the "Plague of Antonious" which struck the Roman Empire somewhere in the period of 164–165 A.D. This epidemic began in the Roman army fighting in Meso-

---

The spread of smallpox to Europe ultimately led to its transfer to the New World by European explorers, conquerors, missionaries, colonists, immigrants, and those engaged in trade, particularly slave trade.

---

potamia and was carried back to Italy by returning soldiers.[7]

Once introduced into Europe, smallpox spread through various channels. Religious movements helped spread the disease. Islamic armies are believed to have brought smallpox from north Africa into Spain, Portugal and France.[8] During the twelfth and thirteenth centuries, the religious crusades to western Asia helped to reintroduce and further spread smallpox in Europe.[9] Smallpox also accompanied armies bent on conquest, merchants following trade routes, and expanding populations. By the fourteenth century, smallpox was well-established in Germany, Spain, Italy, and France.[10] By the latter half of the sixteenth century, smallpox was endemic in most of Europe.[11] The spread of smallpox to Europe ultimately led to its transfer to the New World by European explorers, conquerors, missionaries, colonists, immigrants, and those engaged in trade, particularly slave trade.

The African slaves imported by Europeans to the New World were a major carrier of smallpox. Smallpox was endemic in Africa when Europeans began to explore and colonize the Americas. African slave ships were incubators for disease. Because it was uneconomical to cross the ocean with less than a full load of cargo, captured slaves were frequently held in chains on slave ships for periods of up to 100 days before they left port.[12] In the cramped quarters in which slaves were held, smallpox spread quickly. Slaves with obvious symptoms of the disease were killed and their bodies tossed overboard, so that the ship, upon landing, would appear to have a healthy cargo. Inevitably, however, in a ship exposed to smallpox, some of the slaves who appeared symptom-free upon arrival would develop the disease, spreading it to their New World home.[13]

Smallpox in Central and South America

Columbus is credited with the discovery of the New World; he may also have introduced smallpox to the region. Among the places Columbus explored in 1492 was the island of Hispaniola (now Haiti and the Dominican Republic). It is on this island that the first New World outbreak of smallpox is believed to have occurred.[14] At the time of Columbus' visit, Hispaniola was inhabited by the Taino, the most advanced of the Arawak Indians, a people with a more sophisticated government and religion than any of the other Caribbean peoples.[15] The exact size of the Taino population at the time the

---

> Because smallpox was . . . mainly a childhood
> disease, smallpox epidemics, although deadly, did
> not threaten entire civilizations.

Europeans first encountered them is unknown. Some researchers have estimated that the population was as high as either 3 or 8 million in 1492.[16] One thing we do know is that, in 1496, Columbus' brother Bartolome, who was left on the island while Columbus returned to Spain, authorized a headcount of Indian adults to determine the tribute due the Spanish and came up with a figure of some 1.1 million. This figure ignored significant segments of the population—for example, children under the age of fourteen or the aged—and covered only that half of the island in Spanish control. Extrapolating from Bartholeme's figures, then, the actual population may have been closer to 3 million.[17] Whatever the original population, the next figures we have, which reflect the devastation of smallpox, are truly shocking. In 1507, smallpox, probably brought to Hispaniola by African slaves imported to work in Spanish-owned mines, struck the island.[18] As would be true throughout the New World, smallpox's effect on the indigenous people of Hispaniola was far more devastating than its effect on the Europeans. By 1514, there were only 26,000 surviving Taino. By 1517, only 11,000 remained; and by 1542, there were only 200 Taino on the whole island. Within a decade or two after that, they were extinct.[19]

The reason smallpox was so much more destructive in the New World than in Europe is clear. In Europe, the disease was endemic. As a result, many adults were exposed to smallpox as children, and those that survived had immunity.[20] Because smallpox was, thus, mainly a childhood disease, smallpox epidemics, although deadly, did not threaten entire civilizations. In the New World, by contrast, the entire indigenous population was susceptible to the disease, having no immunity at all. Epidemics which in Europe would kill only the young destroyed large percentages of the entire population in the New World.[21]

Given the absence of immunity among the indigenous New World population, it is no surprise that smallpox's devastation did not stop with the Taino. The disease quickly spread from Hispaniola to other areas in the Caribbean—first to Cuba in 1518 and then to Puerto Rico in 1519, where it killed over half the native population.[22] Having gained a toehold on the three main Spanish-occupied islands, it was inevitable that smallpox would eventually expand with the Spanish explorers to the mainland. A few months after smallpox invaded Cuba, Hernando Cortez sailed from Cuba to Mexico, where he encountered the Aztec civilization and their mighty emperor Montezuma. Montezuma is reported to have greeted the Spaniards warmly at the gates of the Aztec capital, Tenochtitlan. Cortez repaid this kindness with treachery, imprisoning Montezuma and exploiting the Aztecs.[23] The cruelest legacy left by Cortez and the Spanish explorers, however, was smallpox.

The smallpox that struck Mexico struck on a larger scale than previous smallpox invasions. A Franciscan friar, writing in 1541, described one outbreak among the Aztecs:

> when smallpox began to attack the Indians it became so great a pestilence among them throughout the land that in most provinces more than half the population died; in others the proportion was little less. For as the Indians did not know the remedy for the disease and were very much in the habit of bathing frequently, whether well or ill, and continued to do so even when suffering from smallpox, they died in heaps, like bedbugs. Many others died of starvation, because, as they were all taken sick at once, they could not care for each other, nor was there anyone to give them bread or anything else.[24]

Ironically, the spread of the disease that ultimately destroyed the Aztec civilization was facilitated by the very advancements that had made the civilization great. The empire over which Montezuma ruled at the time of Cortez's conquest was huge—stretching from the Gulf of Mexico to the Pacific Ocean and from modern El Salvador to the present-day border of the United States.[25] To control this vast empire, the Aztec rulers had created a network of roads linking all parts of the empire. There was constant travel between the various parts of the Aztec nation.[26] Unfortunately, the roads that linked the Aztec people, and permitted their civilization to flourish, also provided a highway on which smallpox traveled rapidly. Once released in Mexico, smallpox swept through the region unchecked. In two years, between three and four million Indians died of the disease.[27] By 1540, following recurring epidemics, the total native population of Mexico, estimated to have been 11 million at the time of Cortez's arrival, had been reduced to less than 6.5 million. By 1597, it was only 2.5 million.[28]

Following the Aztecs, the next Indian tribes to succumb to smallpox were the native tribes of present-day Guatemala and Honduras. In this case, smallpox pre-

> Smallpox left an indelible mark on Central and South America as a whole.

ceded the Spanish conquistadors as they moved south. The disease struck tribe after tribe, leaving the survivors vulnerable to easy conquest.[29] Eventually, smallpox spread down the Isthmus of Panama through Columbia to Peru where it destroyed another great civilization, that of the Incas. The Spanish explorer Vasco de Balboa had initially discovered the Incan empire during an expedition begun in 1515. He learned that the empire was vast, occupying a territory about the size of the eastern seaboard of present-day United States.[30] In about 1525, the Spanish conquistador Francisco Pizarro set out with a small force of sixty-two horsemen, one-hundred-six footmen, and a few cannon, to conquer and convert the Incas to Spanish rule.[31] He was aided by a powerful ally—smallpox, which appears to have crossed the mountains on foot ahead of him. It devastated the Incan population, killing an estimated 200,000 Indians. One of those killed was the Incan emperor, Huayana Capac. Following Huayana's death, a civil war broke out within the Incan empire. By the time Pizarro arrived in Peru, the civil war and the smallpox epidemic that had helped cause it had created such destruction within the empire that Pizarro was able easily to subdue the Incas.[32] Smallpox had claimed another civilization as its victim. Following the devastation of the Aztecs and the Incas, smallpox continued to spread through Central and South America, sometimes carried by foreign explorers and sometimes carried by the nomadic Indians. By the end of the sixteenth century, smallpox had rampaged through all of Latin America.[33] See attached Appendices.

Consequences of Smallpox for Central and South America

The consequences of smallpox in Central and South America were devastating. Smallpox decimated whole native populations and, with them, their civilizations. Those Indian tribes that survived still saw their populations severely weakened. Religious and political leaders, as well as the community elders, were often lost to the disease. This, in turn, ultimately led to a weakening of the social structure.[34] With the destruction of these extremely advanced civilizations went their ingenuity, their knowledge of their world in which they had lived harmoniously for centuries, and their traditions and cultures.

Apart from its impact on specific populations, smallpox left an indelible mark on Central and South America as a whole, impacting, in fundamental ways, the political, religious, and economic makeup of that region. It was the catalyst that changed the ethnic composition of the region and dictated, to a large extent, the way that blacks and whites would relate to each other for centuries. The transformation began when smallpox devastated the Indian labor pool upon which the Spanish colonists had initially relied to mine the riches of the New World. Forced to import a new labor force to do their work, the Spanish imported large numbers of African slaves.[35] This, in turn, had a number of repercussions for the region: 1) blacks replaced Indians as a major population element of the Western Hemisphere. Today, for example, Jamaica, the Bahamas, Haiti, Cuba and Puerto Rico all have substantial or predominantly black populations in place of the indigenous Indians lost to smallpox[36]; 2) the practice of slavery reached a level of acceptance in the New World not found anywhere else, with long term consequences for the relationship between the black and white populations. Unlike previous instances of forced labor, plantation slavery was defined by race. Moreover, because it was grounded in the idea that black slaves, and their offspring, were inherently and permanently inferior to their white masters, it condemned a whole race to a permanent state of enslavement. The insidious effects of this institutionalized racism would be felt for generations.[37]

Apart from the transformation of the ethnic makeup of the region, and the political and social consequences which followed, smallpox also had a powerful psychological impact on the remaining members of the indigenous populations of Central and South America. As one historian has noted:

> [T]he psychological implications of a disease that killed only Indians and left Spaniards unharmed . . . could only be explained supernaturally, and there could be no doubt about which side of the struggle enjoyed divine favor. the religion, priesthood, and way of life built around the old Indian gods could not survive such a demonstration of the superior power of the God the Spaniards worshipped. Little wonder, then, that the Indians accepted Christianity and submitted to Spanish control so meekly. God had shown Himself on their side . . . [38]

The transformation of the Indian culture caused by smallpox is unique in all of history. In other parts of the world—India, China, and Africa, for example—European imperialism resulted in varying degrees of European political control and the establishment of privileged trade relationships. For the most part, however, the local cultural institutions and religions of the native populations were left intact. This was not the case in Latin America where smallpox magnified the impact of the European presence. As noted by one writer:

Nowhere else, in the history of European imperialism, did an indigenous people surrender religiously as well as politically . . . . Latin America today is dominated by Roman Catholicism and Hispanic culture—a development that could not have taken place without the discrepancy in the immune systems of conquerors and conquered.[39]

Conclusion

One goal of the European colonization effort was to "Europeanize" the newly claimed territory. Besides bringing European plants, animals, and society to the Americas, the Europeans also brought smallpox. Although a strong argument can be made that the European expansion ultimately improved life in the New World, "Europeanizing" the Americas came at a price—the loss of the indigenous peoples who, for centuries, had inhabited the territory, as well as their rich and varied traditions and cultures. Today, the disease that devastated the Incas and the Aztecs no longer theatens mankind and is little more than a footnote in medical textbooks. Nonetheless, its migration to the New World left a mark on the history of that region that can never be erased.

Footnotes

1. Joel N. Shurkin, The Invisible Fire (New York: G.P. Putnam's Sons, 1979), p. 25.

2. G. S. D'Ardois, "La Viruela en la Nueva Espana," in Donald R. Hopkins, Princes and Peasants (Chicago: University of Chicago Press, 1983), p. 206.

3. Zvi Dor-Ner, Columbus and the Age of Discovery (New York: William Morrow and Company, Inc. 1991), p. 216; Hopkins, Princes and Peasants, p. 204. In one of the few surviving Indian writings from the sixteenth century, an elderly Indian, describing the effects of the Spanish conquest, denies the existence of disease in his youth: "There was then no sickness; they had no aching bones; they had then no high fever, then had they no smallpox . . . . At that time the course of humanity was orderly. The foreigners made it otherwise when they arrived here." Book of Chilam Balam of Chumayal, Ralph L. Roy, trans. (Washington, D.C., 1933), p. 83, quoted in Alfred W. Crosby, Jr., "Conquistador y Pestilencia: The First New World Pandemic and the Fall of the Great Indian Empires," Hispanic American Historical Review, 47 (1967), p. 322.

4. Hopkins, p. 15.

5. Ibid., p. 15.

6. Ibid., p. 19.

7. Ibid., p. 22.

8. Ibid., p. 26.

9. Ibid., p. 26.

10. Ibid., p. 28.

11. Ibid., p. 28.

12. Shurkin, pp. 104–05.

13. Ibid., pp. 104–05.

14. Hopkins, p. 204.

15. Dor-Ner, p. 183.

16. Kirkpatrick Sale, The Conquest of Paradise (New York: Alfred A. Knopf Publishing, 1990), p. 161.

17. Sale, p. 160.

18. Hopkins, pp. 204–05.

19. Dor-Ner, p. 218; Sale, p. 161.

20. Indeed this fact may help explain the apparent absence of any serious outbreak of smallpox in the New World for some fifteen years after Columbus' first voyage. As one historian has noted, smallpox "is a deadly malady, but it lasts only a short time in each patient." Crosby, p. 326. Moreover, there is no non-human carrier of smallpox; it must be transmitted from person to person. Most of the early European explorers had probably been exposed to smallpox as children and had at least partial immunity. Given the length of the trans-Atlantic voyage, an isolated individual sailor or immigrant who developed the disease during the journey would either have died of it or recovered from it by the time he landed. In addition, the moist air and strong sunlight experienced on a tropical sea voyage were deadly to the smallpox virus. Thus, it may have taken some time for the smallpox virus to become successfully entrenched in the New World. Ibid., pp. 326–27.

21. Dor-Ner, p. 216; William McNeil, Plagues and Peoples (Garden City: Anchor Press/Doubleday, 1976), p. 208.

22. Shurkin, p. 106.

23. Francis F. Berdan, The Aztecs (New York: Chelsea House Publishers, 1989), pp. 94–98.

24. Elizabeth A. Foster, Motolinia's History of the Indians of New Spain (Berkeley: Cortes Society, 1950), p. 38.

25. Dor-Ner, p. 233.

26. Ibid., p. 233.

27. Shurkin, p. 104.

28. Dor-Ner, p. 235.

29. Shurkin, 106; Hopkins, p. 208.

30. Shurkin, p. 106.

31. Ibid., p. 106.

32. Shurkin, p. 107.

33. Hopkins, p. 212.

34. Dor-Ner, p. 216.

35. Ibid., pp. 227–28; Michael L. Conniff and Thomas J. Davis, Africans in the Americas (New York: St. Martins Press, 1994), p. 74.

36. Dor-Ner, p. 229.

37. Ibid., p. 229.

38. McNeill, p. 2. The submission of the Indians to their Spanish conquerors did not stop with religion. It extended across the board: "Docility to the commands of . . . viceroys, landowners, mining entrepreneurs, tax collectors, and anyone else who spoke with a loud voice and had a white skin was another inevitable consequence [of smallpox]. When the divine and natural orders were both unambiguous in declaring against native tradition and belief, what ground for resistance remained? The extraordinary ease of Spanish conquests and the success a few hundred men had in securing control of vast areas and millions of persons is unintelligible on any other basis." Ibid., p. 208.

39. Dor-Ner, p. 234.

Annotated Bibliography

Primary Sources

D'Ardois, G.S. "La Viruela en la Nueva Espana." Gac. Med. Mex. 91 (1961): 1015–24, translated and quoted in Hopkins, Donald R. Princes and Peasants. Chicago: University of Chicago Press, 1983.

A translation of parts of a diary compiled by a Franciscan friar in the six-teenth century detailing his life with the Indians of what is present-day Mexico. Contains a graphic description of the effects of smallpox on the native population.

De Fuentes, Patricia. The Conquistadors. New York: Orion, 1963.

Translations of first person accounts of various Spanish explorers, includ-ing Hernando Cortez. Good discussion of the conquest of the Aztecs from the perspective of the Spaniards. Although the accounts do not explicitly mention smallpox, they do describe the deaths of thousands of the Aztec Indians as a result of a disease whose description suggests that it may have been smallpox.

Foster, Elizabeth A. Motolinia's History of the Indians of New Spain. Ber-keley: Cortes Society, 1950.

A translation of parts of the diary of Fray Toribio Motolinia, a Francisan friar, describing life among the Indians of Mexico. Contains excellent discussion of smallpox's impact on the Indians.

Hemming, John. Red Gold. Cambridge: Harvard University Press, 1978.

This book describes the Spanish conquest of present day Brazil. Although the book was written in the 1900s, and, therefore, appears to be a sec-ondary source, it contains extensive translations of primary source doc-uments, including letters and diaries, written in the sixteenth century.

Moses, Bernard. The Spanish Dependencies in South America. New York: Harper and Brothers, 1914.

A book consisting largely of primary source material describing the devel-opment of the Spanish colonies in South America. Several of the pri-mary source translations describe the devastating effects of smallpox on the Incas.

Berdan, Francis F. The Aztecs. New York: Chelsea House Publishers, 1989.

History of the Aztec civilization, including discussion of its destruction at the hands of the Spaniards and the role of smallpox in that destruc-tion.

Conniff, Michael L. and Thomas J. Davis. Africans in the Americas. New York: St. Martins Press, 1994.

History of the African migration to the Americas including a discussion of the early slave trade and its impact on the Caribbean region.

Crosby, A.W. "Conquistador y Pestilencia: The First New World Pandemic and the Fall of the Great Indian Empires." Hispanic American Histori-cal Review (1967) 47: 321–27.

Well-documented and detailed analysis of the smallpox epidemics that brought down the Aztec and Incan civilizations. Contains excerpts from primary source material.

Crow, John A. The Epic of Latin America. Garden City: Doubleday, 1971.

A long (900 page) treatise discussing the history of Latin America with extensive discussion of the early Spanish exploration. Contains only brief discussion of smallpox. However, this source provides an excellent background discussion of the early Spanish conquests, including the conquests of the Incas and the Aztecs.

Dobyns, H.G. "An Outline of Andean Epidemic History to 1720." Bulletin of the History of Medicine (1963) 37: 493–515.
Paper discussing, among other things, the smallpox epidemics that preceded and lead up to the collapse of the Incan empire.
Dor-Ner, Zvi. Columbus and the Age of Discovery. New York: William Morrow and Company, Inc., 1991.
A description of the voyages of Columbus to the New World and the historical impact of those voyages, including a discussion of the historical consequences of smallpox in the New World.
Helps, Arthur. The Spanish Conquest of America. London: John Lane, 1904.
Multi-volume treatise looking, as the name suggests, at the Spanish conquest of Central and South America. Contains excerpts from primary source materials.
Hopkins, Donald R. Princes and Peasants. Chicago: University of Chicago Press, 1983.
A very extensive discussion of the history of smallpox from its inception to the last reported cases worldwide. Contains excerpts from primary source material.
McNeill, William A. Plagues and Peoples. Garden City: Anchor Press/Doubleday, 1976.
This book examines the impact of disease on people and civilizations throughout history. One chapter is devoted exclusively to the devastating effects of smallpox on the Aztec and Incan cultures.
Sale, Kirkpatrick. The Conquest of Paradise. New York: Alfred A. Knopf Publishing, 1990.
Discussion of the early European exploration of the New World. Contains a good description of the effect of smallpox on the Taino Indian tribe. Also contains excerpts from primary source material.
Shurkin, Joel N. The Invisible Fire. New York: G.P. Putnam's Sons, 1979.
An extremely helpful book describing the search for a cure for smallpox. Contains a good discussion of the effect of smallpox on Central and South America. Also contains excerpts from primary source material.

Appendix I: Smallpox's Migration Through Central America

1518—Hernando Cortez sails from Cuba to Mexico; arrives at Aztec capital of Tenochtitlan in November 1519. (Hopkins, 205)

1519—Governor of Cuba, who sent Cortez to Mexico, becomes suspicious of Cortez' loyalty and sends another expedition led by Panfilo de Narvaez to Mexico with orders to supersede Cortez. (Hopkins, 205)

1520—Narvaez lands at Cempoala, near present-day Vera Cruz in April. According to a number of historians, it was an African slave in Narvaez's party that first introduced smallpox to the American mainland. (Hopkins, 205)

Summer 1520—smallpox spreads to the edge of Mexico's inland plateau. In September, it reaches towns around the lakes in the Valley of Mexico (near present day Mexico City). In September or October, it invades Aztec capital of Tenochtitlan. (Hopkins, 205)

Fall of 1520—Smallpox claims the life of Montezuma's successor Cuitlahuac. (Helps, 2:301)

1520—Cortez is forced to retreat from Tenochtitlan to Tlascala, a stronghold of the Spaniards' Indian allies. There, he learns of the death from smallpox of a local ruler Maxixca. The head of another of the Aztec provinces (Chalco Province) also dies of smallpox at about this time. In these, and other instances, Cortez is able to solidify the Spaniards' position with the local Indians by taking a leadership role in settling disputes about the succession of new rulers and ensuring that chiefs friendly to the Spanish conquerors are installed in place of those killed by smallpox. (Hopkins, 207)

  The importance of the smallpox epidemic as a factor in the success of the Spanish conquest is confirmed in the comments of one soldier traveling with Cortez: "When the Christians were exhausted from war, God saw fit to send the Indians smallpox, and there was a great pestilence in the city . . . . We soldiers could scarcely get about the streets because of the Indians who were sick from hunger, pestilence and smallpox. Also for these reasons they began to slacken in their fighting." (de Fuentes, 159) (diary of Francisco deAguilar). The smallpox epidemic gives a weary Cortez an opportunity to regroup and marshal more Indian allies. In May 1521, he returns to Tenochtitlan and captures the Aztec capital three months later. (Hopkins, 207)

1523—Smallpox travels south. By the time the Spanish begin to push into Mayan territory, smallpox has preceded them, destroying large numbers of the Indian population in Guatemala and the Yucatan. In these areas, smallpox outbreaks in 1520 and 1521 "carried off half the Cakchiquel population, including two rulers, and greatly decreased the formerly thick population in the northern interior of the Yucatecan Peninsula." (Dobyns, 495–96). The Mayans call this plague nohkakil, meaning the "Great Fire." (Hopkins, 208)

APPENDIX II: SMALLPOX'S MIGRATION THROUGH SOUTH AMERICA

1587—Smallpox epidemic in Colombia kills 90% of the Indians around Bogota (Hopkins, 213)

1533, 1558, 1580 and 1586—smallpox epidemics ravage Ecuador (Hopkins, 212).

1524—smallpox epidemic devastates the Inca empire, leaving it vulnerable to conquest by Spanish conquistador Francisco Pizarro (Hopkins, 208).

1580—Portuguese ship imports smallpox into Venezuela in 1580; epidemic destroys entire tribes of Indians. (Hopkins, 213)

1560's—smallpox carried inland to the forests of Brazil by terrified Indians trying to escape the infection on the coast. Jesuit missionaries unwittingly contribute to devastation of natives by herding them into mission settlements ostensibly as a means of protecting them from epidemics that had ravaged coastal areas. (Hopkins, 215)

1533, 1535, 1558, 1587—smallpox outbreaks in Peru. One witness to the 1585 outbreak describes devastation as follows: "They died in scores and hundreds. Villages were depopulated. Corpses were scattered over the fields or piled up in the houses or huts. All branches of industrial activity were paralyzed. The fields were uncultivated; the herds were untended; and the workshops and the mines were without laborers. It was only with difficulty that the ships could be manned. The price of food rose to such an extent that many persons found it beyond their reach. They escaped the foul disease, but only to be wasted by famine." (Moses 1914, 1:385).

1554—Spanish soldiers introduce smallpox into Chile; one writer describes impact in one district, stating that of the twelve thousand people who originally lived in the region, "not more than a hundred escaped with life." (Hopkins, 213)

1603—slave ships introduce smallpox into Buenos Aires. (Hopkins, 216)

1555—French Huguenots carry smallpox to Brazil while establishing settlement near present day Rio de Janeiro. Five years later, African slaves reintroduce smallpox to Brazil (Hopkins, 214)

1563—Portuguese ship introduces smallpox into Ilheus in Brazil; epidemic spreads to Bahia, killing between one-fourth and two-thirds of those it encounters (Hopkins, 214). A letter from a Portuguese resident of Bahia written in 1563 describes the epidemic: "This was a form of smallpox or pox so loathsome and evil-smelling that none could stand the great stench that emerged from them. For this reason many died untended, consumed by the worms that grew in the wounds of the pox and were engendered in their bodies in such abundance and of such great size that they caused horror and shock to any who saw them." (Hopkins, 214)

Sick City

Maps and Mortality in the Time of Cholera

BY STEVEN SHAPIN
THE NEW YORKER, NOVEMBER 6, 2006

After Katrina, cholera. On August 31, 2005—two days after the hurricane made landfall—the Bush Administration's Health and Human Services Secretary warned, "We are gravely concerned about the potential for cholera, typhoid, and dehydrating diseases that could come as a result of the stagnant water and other conditions." Around the world, newspapers and other media evoked the spectre of cholera in the United States, the world's hygienic superpower. A newspaper in Columbus, Ohio, reported that New Orleans was a cesspool of "enough cholera germs to wipe out Los Angeles." And a paper in Tennessee, where some New Orleans refugees had arrived, whipped up fear among the locals with the headline "KATRINA EVACUEE DIAGNOSED WITH CHOLERA."

There was to be no outbreak of cholera in New Orleans, nor among the residents who fled. Despite raw sewage and decomposing bodies floating in the toxic brew that drowned the city, cholera was never likely to happen: there was little evidence that the specific bacteria that cause cholera were present. But the point had been made: Katrina had reduced a great American city to Third World conditions. Twenty-first-century America had had a cholera scare.

Cholera is a horrific illness. The onset of the disease is typically quick and spectacular; you can be healthy one moment and dead within hours. The disease, left untreated, has a fatality rate that can reach fifty per cent. The first sign that you have it is a sudden and explosive watery diarrhea, classically described as "rice-water stool," resembling the water in which rice has been rinsed and sometimes having a fishy smell. White specks floating in the stool are bits of lining from the small intestine. As a result of water loss—vomiting often accompanies diarrhea, and as much as a litre of water may be lost per hour—your eyes become sunken; your body is racked with agonizing cramps; the skin becomes leathery; lips and face turn blue; blood pressure drops; heartbeat becomes irregular; the amount of oxygen reaching your cells diminishes. Once you enter hypovolemic shock, death can follow within minutes. A mid-nineteenth-century English newspaper report described cholera victims who were "one minute warm, palpitating, human organisms—the next a sort of galvanized corpse, with icy breath, stopped

pulse, and blood congealed—blue, shrivelled up, convulsed."
Through it all, and until the very last stages, is the added horror of
full consciousness. You are aware of what's happening: "the mind
within remains untouched and clear,—shining strangely through
the glazed eyes . . . a spirit, looking out in terror from a corpse."

You may know precisely what is going to happen to you because
cholera is an epidemic disease, and unless you are fortunate enough
to be the first victim you have probably seen many others die of it,
possibly members of your own family, since the disease often affects
households en bloc. Once cholera begins, it can spread with terrifying speed. Residents of cities in its path used to track cholera's
approach in the daily papers, panic growing as nearby cities were
struck. Those who have the means to flee do, and the refugees cause
panic in the places to which they've fled. Writing from Paris during
the 1831–32 epidemic, the poet Heinrich Heine said that it "was as
if the end of the world had come." The people fell on the victims "like
beasts, like maniacs."

Cholera is now remarkably easy to treat: the key is to quickly provide victims with large amounts of fluids and electrolytes.

Cholera is now remarkably easy to treat: the key is to quickly provide victims with large amounts of fluids and electrolytes. That simple regime can reduce the fatality rate to less than one per cent. In
2004, there were only five cases of cholera reported to the Centers
for Disease Control, four of which were acquired outside the U.S.,
and none of which proved fatal. Epidemic cholera is now almost
exclusively a Third World illness—often appearing in the wake of
civil wars and natural disasters—and it is a major killer only in
places lacking the infrastructure for effective emergency treatment.
Within the last several years, there has been cholera in Angola,
Sudan (including Darfur), the Democratic Republic of the Congo,
and an arc of West African countries from Senegal to Niger. In the
early nineteen-nineties, there were more than a million cases in
Latin America, mass deaths from cholera among the refugees from
Rwandan genocide in 1994, and regular outbreaks in India and
Bangladesh, especially after floods. The World Health Organization
calls cholera "one of the key indicators of social development." Its
presence is a sure sign that people are not living with civilized
amenities.

Cholera is caused by a comma-shaped bacterium—*Vibrio cholerae*—whose role was identified by the German physician Robert
Koch in 1883. By far the most common route of infection is drinking
contaminated water. And, since water comes to contain *V. cholerae*
through the excrement of cholera victims, an outbreak of the disease
is evidence that people have been drinking each other's feces. Much

of modern civilization has been geared toward making sure that this doesn't happen. One reason is simply that it's disgusting, but another reason is that it puts us at risk of cholera—a discovery owing largely to the work of a mid-nineteenth-century English doctor named John Snow. His work is celebrated in Steven Johnson's vivid history "The Ghost Map: The Story of London's Most Terrifying Epidemic—and How It Changed Science, Cities, and the Modern World" (Riverhead; $26.95). Snow didn't know about *V. cholerae*, but identifying contaminated water as the vehicle of transmission has made him one of medical history's heroes.

The word "cholera" derives from *choler*—the Greek word for yellow bile—perhaps because of the pale appearance of the resulting evacuations. Hippocrates mentioned cholera as a common post-childhood disease, but given that he thought it might be brought on by eating goat's meat he was probably referring to a less malign form of diarrhea. It was almost certainly not the life-threatening epidemic disease that emerged from India in 1817 and which then began its spread around the world, travelling, as Snow said, "along the great tracks of human intercourse"—colonialism and global trade. The first pandemic of what the British and the Americans called Asiatic cholera (or cholera morbus) reached Southeast Asia, East Africa, the Middle East, and the Caucasus, but petered out in 1823. A second pandemic, between 1826 and 1837, also originated in India, but this time it took a devastating toll on both Europe and America, arriving in Britain in the autumn of 1831 and in America the following year. By 1833, twenty thousand people had died of cholera in England and Wales, with London especially hard hit. A third pandemic swept England and Wales in 1848–49 (more than fifty thousand dead) and again in 1854, when thirty thousand died in London alone.

At the time, the idea that cholera might be transmitted by a waterborne poison ran against the grain of medical opinion. Disease was not generally viewed as a "thing"—a specific pathological entity caused by a specific external agency. Instead, it was common to suppose that diseases reflected an imbalance of the four humors (blood, phlegm, and yellow and black bile), an imbalance ascribed to a large range of behaviors and environmental factors. Moreover, epidemic disease—literally, disease coming "upon the people"—was then widely ascribed not to contagion but to atmospheric "miasmas." In the seventeenth century, the great English physician Thomas Sydenham had introduced the notion of an "epidemic constitution of the atmosphere." Something had contaminated the local air (possibly, he thought, noxious effluvia from "the bowels of the earth") in a way that unbalanced the humors. The occasional appearance of these effluvia accounted for the intermittent character of epidemic disease. The miasmal theory remained medical orthodoxy for about two centuries. (We owe to it the name of the disease malaria: literally, "bad air.") In mid-nineteenth-century usage, a disease was called "epidemic" if it was *not* thought to be "contagious."

The fact that the poor suffered most in many epidemics was readily accommodated by the miasmal theory: certain people—those who lived in areas where the atmosphere was manifestly contaminated and who led a filthy and unwholesome way of life—were "predisposed" to be afflicted. The key indicator of miasma was stench. An aphorism of the nineteenth-century English sanitary reformer Edwin Chadwick was "All smell is disease." Sydenham's belief in a subterranean origin of miasmas gradually gave way to the view that they were caused by the accumulation of putrefying organic materials—a matter of human responsibility. As Charles E. Rosenberg's hugely influential work "The Cholera Years" (1962) noted, when Asiatic cholera first made its appearance in the United States, in 1832, "Medical opinion was unanimous in agreeing that the intemperate, the imprudent, the filthy were particularly vulnerable." During an early outbreak in the notorious Five Points neighborhood of Manhattan, a local newspaper maintained that this was an area inhabited by the most wretched specimens of humanity: "Be the air pure from Heaven, their breath would contaminate it, and infect it with disease." The map of cholera seemed so intimately molded to the moral order that, as Rosenberg put it, "to die of cholera was to die in suspicious circumstances." Rather like syphilis, it was taken as a sign that you had lived in a way you ought not to have lived. "The great mass of people . . . don't know that the miasma of an unscavenged street or impure alley is productive of cholera and disease," the English liberal economic activist Richard Cobden observed in 1853. "If they did know these things, people would take care that they inhabited better houses."

Élite presumptions to the contrary, the London poor did not enjoy living in squalor. In 1849, a group of them wrote a joint letter to the London *Times*:

> We live in muck and filthe. We aint got no priviz, no dust bins, no drains, no water-splies . . . . The Stenche of a Gully-hole is disgustin. We all of us suffer, and numbers are ill, and if the Colera comes Lord help us. . . . We are livin like piggs, and it aint faire we shoulde be so ill treted.

But some sanitary reformers, Florence Nightingale among them, opposed contagionism precisely because they believed that the poor were personally responsible for their filth: contagionism undermined your ability to hold people to account for their unwholesome way of life. Whereas, in a miasmal view of the world, the distribution of disease followed the contours of morality—your nose just knew it—infection by an external agent smacked of moral randomness.

What to do? In the middle of the nineteenth century, there was a host of nostrums for sale. In fashionable Paris, people put their faith in flannel: *Le Figaro* proclaimed, "Today, Venus would wear a flannel girdle," and Heine added, "The King, too, now wears a belly-band of the best bourgeois flannel." Another popular preventative was to surround yourself with camphor vapors to counteract the noxious smell, and still another was to smother your food with garlic. On a neighborhood scale, you might achieve the same effect by burning tar, pitch, sugar, or vinegar, or by liberal use of chloride of lime in the home and on the streets, its bleachy smell giving olfactory assurance that the miasmas had been effectively countered. On a municipal level, one of the most important courses of action was to empty out the thousands of back-yard cesspools in which household excrement was kept and which periodically overflowed and ran down the streets in brown, reeking rivers. You could also pray: insofar as cholera was a divine scourge, you could supplement a renewed dedication to God's laws of wholesome living by beseeching divine benevolence. Days of prayer, fasting, and humiliation were decreed. A calm and pious state of mind was recommended. Temperate feeding and drinking were prescribed; debauchery was contraindicated. Moderation in these things was not only good morality; it was good medicine. In the 1832 outbreak, many New Yorkers reassured themselves that the only countries that had yet suffered grievously were heathen: Christian America would surely not be hard punished.

When cholera hit London in 1848, John Snow was well placed to doubt the miasmal theory. A founding member of the London Epidemiological Society, Snow was also an anesthetist—administering gas to Queen Victoria at the first chloroform-assisted royal birth—and he had made a study of gaseous diffusion. Why was it, he wondered, that people most exposed to these supposedly noxious miasmas—sewer workers, for example—were no more likely to be afflicted with cholera than anyone else? Snow also knew that the concentration of gases declined rapidly over distance, so how could a miasma arising from one source pollute the atmosphere of a whole neighborhood, or even a city? Why, if many of those closest to the stench were unaffected, did some of those far removed from it become ill? And there were some notable outbreaks of cholera that didn't appear to fit with the moral and evidential underpinnings of miasmal theory. Sometimes the occupants of one building fell ill while those in an adjacent building, at least as squalid, escaped. Moreover, cholera attacked the alimentary, not the respiratory, tract. Why should that be, if the vehicle of contagion was in the air as opposed to something ingested?

Snow's attempt to make sense of these observations, in the years after the 1848 epidemic, led him to the water supply. He began to look at the physical networks by which London's neighborhoods were served with water. By the middle of the nineteenth century, the municipal supply was a hodgepodge of ancient and more modern history. From medieval times, water had been drawn both from urban wells and from the Thames and its tributaries. In the early seventeenth century, the so-called New River was constructed; it carried Hertfordshire spring water, by gravity alone, to Clerkenwell, a distance of almost forty miles. During the eighteenth century and the early nineteenth, a number of private water companies were established, taking water from the Thames and using newly invented steam pumps to deliver it by iron pipe. By the middle of the nineteenth century, there were about ten companies supplying London's water. Many of these companies drew their water from within the Thames's tidal section, where the city's sewage was also dumped, thus providing customers with excrement-contaminated drinking water. In the early eighteen-fifties, Parliament had ordered the water companies to shift their intake pipes above the tideway by August of 1855: some complied quickly; others dragged their feet.

When cholera returned, in 1854, Snow was able to identify a number of small districts served by two water companies, one still supplying a fecal cocktail and one that had moved its intake pipes to Thames Ditton, above the tidal section. Snow compiled tables showing a strong connection in these districts between cholera mortality and water source. Snow's "grand experiment" was supposed to be decisive: there were no pertinent variables distinguishing the two populations other than the origins of their drinking water. As it turned out, the critical evidence came not from this study of commercially piped river water but from a fine-grained map showing the roles of different wells. Snow lived on Sackville Street, just around the corner from the Royal Academy of Arts, and in late August cholera erupted practically next door, in an area of Soho. It was, Snow later wrote, "the most terrible outbreak of cholera which ever occurred in this kingdom"—more than five hundred deaths in ten days.

Snow now had the theory and the statistics to chart this epidemic and to establish its waterborne cause. Using the *Weekly Return of Births and Deaths*, which was published by William Farr, a statistician in the Office of the Registrar-General, and a staunch anti-contagionist, Snow homed in on the microstructure of the epidemic. He began to suspect contaminated water in a well on Broad Street whose pump served households in about a two-block radius. The well had nothing to do with commercially piped water—which in this neighborhood happened to be relatively pure—but it was suspicious nonetheless. Scientists at the time knew no more about the invisible constituents of the water supply than they did about the attributes of specific miasmas—Snow wrote that the "morbid poison" of cholera "must necessarily have some sort of structure, most likely that of a cell," but he could not see anything that looked relevant under the microscope—so even Snow still used smell as an important diagnostic sign. He recorded a local impression that, at the height of the outbreak, the Broad Street well water had an atypically "offensive smell," and that those who were deterred by it from drinking the water did not fall ill. What Snow needed was not the biological or chemical identity of the "morbid poison," or formal proof of causation, but a powerful rhetoric of persuasion. The map

Snow produced, in 1854, plotted cholera mortality house by house in the affected area, with bars at each address that showed the number of dead. The closer you lived to the Broad Street pump, the higher the pile of bars. A few streets away, around the pump at the top of Carnaby Street, there were scarcely any bars, and slightly farther, near the Warwick Street pump, there were none at all.

The map occupies a deservedly prominent place in Edward R. Tufte's 1983 masterpiece "The Visual Display of Quantitative Information," but it was not in itself decisive. Suppose that the cholera-causing miasmas were just concentrated that way? But Snow's study of the neighborhood enabled him to add persuasive anecdotal evidence to the anonymity of statistics. Just across from the Broad Street pump was the Poland Street workhouse, whose wretched inmates, living closely packed in miserable conditions, should have been ideal cholera victims. Yet the disease scarcely touched them. The workhouse, it emerged, had its own well and a piped supply from a company with uncontaminated Thames water. Similarly, there were no cholera deaths among the seventy workers in the Lion Brewery, on Broad Street. They drank mainly malt liquor, and the brewery had its own well. What Snow called the "most conclusive" evidence concerned a widow living far away, in salubrious Hampstead, and her niece, who lived in "a high and healthy part of Islington": neither had gone anywhere near Broad Street, and both succumbed to cholera within days of its Soho outbreak. It turned out that the widow used to live in the affected area, and had developed a taste for the Broad Street well water. She had secured a supply on August 31st, and, when her niece visited, both drank from the same deadly bottle.

Next, Snow had to show how the Broad Street well had got infected, and for this he made use of the detailed knowledge of a local minister, Henry Whitehead. The minister had at first been skeptical of Snow's waterborne theories, but became convinced by the evidence the doctor was gathering. Whitehead discovered that the first, or "index," case of the Soho cholera was a child living on Broad Street: her diapers had been rinsed in water that was then tipped into a cesspool in front of a house just a few feet away from the well. The cesspool leaked and so, apparently, did the well. Snow persuaded the parish Board of Guardians to remove the handle from the Broad Street pump, pretty much ending the Soho cholera outbreak. There's now a replica of the handleless pump outside a nearby pub named in John Snow's honor.

Johnson is aware that Snow's victory was not instantaneous or uncontested. Neither the medical community nor policymakers were immediately convinced. For all Snow's wisdom, dedication, and intellectual originality, the parish board that removed the pump handle did not specifically accept his theory. The national Board of Health saw "no reason" to fall in with Snow; and the miasmal theory was flexible enough to accommodate even some of his purportedly crucial evidence. (Suppose, for example, that poisons in the atmosphere were what infected the Broad Street water.) Johnson calls this "circular argumentation at its most devious," and, of course, in retrospect, the Board of Health was wrong. But attempting to save a scientific theory that seemed so well supported, and that had survived for so long, is neither as irrational as outside commentators suppose nor as historically rare as they would like.

Snow gradually gained more supporters, but the major public-health reforms of the ensuing years were not direct results of his work, and some were even inspired by the miasmal theory that he did so much to combat. In the oppressively hot summer of 1858, London was overwhelmed by what the papers called "the Great Stink." The already sewage-loaded Thames had begun to carry the additional burden of thousands of newly invented flush water closets, and improved domestic sanitation was producing the paradoxical result of worsened public sanitation. The Thames had often reeked before, but this time politicians fled the Houses of Parliament, on the river's embankment, or attended with handkerchiefs pressed to their noses. "Whoso once inhales the stink can never forget it," a newspaper reported, "and can count himself lucky if he live to remember it." Measures to clean up the Thames had been on the agenda for some years, but an urgent fear of miasmas broke a political logjam, and gave immediate impetus to one of the great monuments of Victorian civil engineering: Sir Joseph Bazalgette's system of municipal sewers, designed to deposit London's waste below the city and far from the intakes of its water supply. (The system became fully operational in the mid-eighteen-seventies, and its pipes and pumps continue to serve London today.)

In the event, the Great Stink's effects on municipal health were negligible: the *Weekly Return* showed no increase in deaths from epidemic disease, confounding miasmatists' expectations. When cholera returned to London in 1866, its toll was much smaller, and the main outbreak was traced to a section of Bazalgette's system which had yet to be completed. In many people's opinion, Snow, who had died in 1858, now stood vindicated. And yet the improved municipal water system that rid the city of cholera had been promoted by sanitary reformers who held to the miasmal theory of disease—people who believed that sewage-laden drinking water was only a minor source of miasmas, but disgusting all the same. The right things were done, but not necessarily for the right scientific reasons.

The brilliance of Snow's map lay, as Johnson argues, in the way that it layered knowledge of different scales—from a bird's-eye view of the structure of the Soho neighborhood to the aggregated mortality statistics printed in the *Weekly Return* to the location of neighborhood water supplies—all framed by particular understandings of how people tended to move about in the neighborhood, of the physical proximity of particular cesspools to particular wells, and of the likely behavior of specific, still invisible, and still unnamed pathogens. A city is a concentration of knowledge as much as it is a concentration of people, buildings, thoroughfares, pipes, and bacteria. Maps like Snow's allowed the modern city to remake itself and to understand itself in a new way. They collected different sorts of knowledge, represented them vividly on the scale of a tabletop, and made that representation available as a resource for urban reform: a plan and a plan of action. If Snow's theory was not the major cause of Victorian sanitary reforms, maps like his were certainly one element in a historical revolution in urban living and in how our culture came to think about urban life: no longer subject to the caprices of divine will but a human environment whose well-being was in the care of human institutions and the expert knowledge contained within those institutions; no longer a pustulating excrescence on the divinely ordained pastoral order—"the Great Wen," as William Cobbett called London—but the natural habitat for humankind, teeming, sociable, and now, at last, healthy. Modern medical theory helped bring about that state of affairs, but so did a more diffuse sense of what it means to live in a civilized state.

Of course, this is a state that continues to elude much of the world—including all those underdeveloped countries which are currently experiencing what epidemiologists call the Seventh Pandemic. The problem is no longer an incorrect understanding of the cause: around the world, people have known for more than a century what you have to do to prevent cholera. Rather, cholera persists because of infrastructural inadequacies that arise from such social and political circumstances as the Third World's foreign-debt burdens, inequitable world-trade regimes, local failures of urban planning, corruption, crime, and incompetence. Victorian London illustrates how much could be done with bad science; the continuing existence of cholera in the Third World shows that even good science is impotent without the resources, the institutions, and the will to act.

Flu's Worst Season

By Nell Boyce
U.S. News & World Report, August 12, 2002

Five years ago, when scientists at the Armed Forces Institute of Pathology announced that they had recovered genes from the infamous 1918 flu virus, they hoped to make quick progress toward explaining an epidemic that killed some 50 million people. The genes had lurked in tissue saved from two soldiers who died of flu and in the body of an Inuit woman buried in permafrost. So far, however, researchers have sequenced five of the virus's eight genes without finding an obvious "smoking gun" that would explain its toll. Jeffrey Taubenberger, one of the team members, calls it "a very ordinary-looking virus."

Last week, however, Taubenberger and a team led by Adolfo Garcia-Sastre at Mount Sinai School of Medicine in New York announced the first hint of something exceptional. They found that adding one of the 1918 genes to a lab flu strain enhanced its ability to block a key immune system response, suggesting the 1918 flu may have been able to partially disarm the body's defenses. The result, published online by the Proceedings of the National Academy of Sciences, is just the start of an explanation for the 1918 pandemic. But it's a "very interesting" one, says flu expert Yoshihiro Kawaoka of the University of Wisconsin-Madison.

The first genetic studies of the 1918 virus focused on genes for surface proteins, where changes can give the virus a new look and allow it to evade the immune system. In the smaller pandemics of 1957 and 1968, the flu took off because it nabbed a surface-protein gene from bird influenza, catching its victims' immune systems by surprise. In the 1918 virus, however, that gene looked more mammalian than birdlike—judging by today's bird flus, anyway. Bird flu might have looked different decades ago. So scientists recently hunted through a Smithsonian Institution collection of wild birds from 1917. They found one goose with the virus—and it looks like today's bird virus, exonerating a newly acquired bird gene, they say in the August Journal of Virology.

Since the 1918 flu didn't seem to emerge in the usual way, scientists have turned to other genes, coding for internal proteins. The gene in the latest study initially looked innocent when the researchers put it into a flu virus and tested it in mice, perhaps because of the species difference. But then they infected a dish of human lung cells and used a "gene chip" to analyze the response of 13,000 different cellular genes. One change stood out: The 1918 gene seemed to stifle some genes normally turned on by interferons, compounds that rally immune defenses.

Reviving a Virus

The team next plans to use this system to test viruses equipped with other 1918 genes. They're also searching for flu in lung tissue from people who died from 1900 to 1918, hoping to pinpoint subtle changes that may have occurred just before the epidemic. Eventually, flu experts hope to reconstruct the entire 1918 virus and—in highly secure labs—test it against animals to learn its secrets. If scientists could figure out 1918, they could help public health workers detect emerging strains with pandemic potential.

But would they also aid would-be bioterrorists? Taubenberger doesn't think hard-to-control flu viruses would make attractive weapons. And he suspects the viral genes probably interact in unknown ways to make a pandemic: "You couldn't just say, 'I'm going to design a really nasty virus' and make it. We just don't understand the rules yet."

Although mixing and matching genes might someday make a bad flu, a 1918-scale pandemic might take something more. Three flu genes are left to sequence, but experts increasingly think genes won't tell the whole story. Part of what made the 1918 virus deadly may have been the people it infected. Strangely, the epidemic killed unusually large numbers of 20-to-35-year-olds—even though flu normally kills the elderly. Could something about young people's immune systems have set them up to be especially hard hit? As Taubenberger's colleague Ann Reid recently put it, "I don't think we can say we have answered the question of what made the 1918 flu so virulent unless we can explain this."

Conquering Polio

By Renee Skelton

National Geographic World, May 2000

Summer was a time of fear in the early 1900s. Warm weather usually meant the annual return of a terrifying disease with the power to disable or even kill. It swept through town after town, mostly attacking small children. Victims might complain of headaches or runny noses. Sometimes these symptoms just disappeared after a day or two, but often they worsened. Leg stiffness and weakened muscles set in. Finally victims could become paralyzed, or unable to move parts of their bodies. Sometimes they died.

The disease was poliomyelitis (poe-lee-oh-my-uh-LYE-tuhs), or polio for short. The first large polio epidemic in the United States occurred in 1916. By year's end, 6,000 people had died and 27,000, mostly children, were paralyzed. At the peak of the polio epidemics in 1952, 58,000 Americans were stricken.

"People had no experience with the disease," says Jane S. Smith, a polio historian. "It came from nowhere and couldn't be prevented in any way people knew. There was a sense of helplessness."

Why did polio strike children more often than adults? How did scientists eventually stop this disease? Read on to find out.

Until the 1900s serious polio cases were rare, and polio epidemics were almost unknown. This puzzled health experts, who also wondered why polio, suddenly widespread, seemed most severe in the wealthiest countries. They found out that a new emphasis on sanitation in these countries was a problem.

Uncovering the Truth

The polio virus spreads through contact with body waste from people carrying the disease. It enters the body through the mouth and moves into the intestines. The virus can continue to the central nervous system, where it damages or destroys nerve tissue. Even people who show mild symptoms, or no symptoms, can pass the disease to others.

Before modern sanitation and plumbing improvements, most infants were exposed to the polio virus. Still protected by antibodies, or proteins that fight disease, they received from their mothers' bodies before they were born, the infants got a mild flu-like form of polio. As a result of that early exposure, their bodies then contained polio antibodies that gave most children lifetime immunity.

FROM PARALYSIS TO PREVENTION

1500 B.C.

Artifacts show that polio was present in ancient times. Archaeologists digging in Egypt near the Nile River in the early 20th century find a mummy with a leg that was probably withered by the disease.

1916

The first polio epidemic occurs in the United States, causing panic. The homes of polio victims are marked with quarantine signs, on the left, to warn people. Residents must stay inside.

1938

The National Foundation for Infantile Paralysis launches the "March of Dimes" campaign to raise money for polio patient care and research. People donate two million dollars to combat polio, also called infantile paralysis.

1949

After several years of research, three scientists discover how to grow the polio virus. In 1955 Jonas Salk develops a killed-virus vaccine that can prevent polio.

1961

Albert Sabin's livevirus vaccine is approved in the U.S. Sabin's vaccine, taken by mouth, soon replaces Salk's injected vaccine.

2000

An effective vaccine makes "wild" polio—polio spread by an infected person—a thing of the past in the United States and most other countries. But polio remains a problem in some countries in Africa, Asia, and the Middle East, where there is little money for health services or where war prevents distribution of vaccines. Health experts hope that immunization will wipe out polio worldwide by the end of 2000.

The sanitation improvements of the 20th century meant that babies were rarely exposed to the polio virus. So their bodies did not build up the immunity necessary to fight the disease. When exposed to the polio virus later in life, these children often got a serious form of the disease.

During the late 1700s and 1800s, researchers successfully created vaccines for smallpox and other diseases. A vaccine is a weakened or killed form of a virus. Its presence in someone's body is enough to trigger the production of antibodies, but rarely causes the disease.

The Search for Prevention

At the height of the polio epidemics during the 1950s, doctors Jonas Salk and Albert Sabin were at work on two different kinds of polio vaccine. Salk used killed–polio virus in his research. He developed an effective vaccine in 1954 and tested it on 1.8 million schoolchildren. In 1955 a relieved nation learned of the vaccine's success.

The number of cases of polio dropped dramatically after the Salk vaccine became widely used. But many scientists, including Sabin, believed that only a vaccine made with weakened live virus would give long-lasting and widespread immunity to polio. They thought those immunized with the Salk vaccine might still spread the disease.

In 1961 the Sabin polio vaccine was approved for use in the U.S. For 40 years Sabin's vaccine replaced Salk's. Today scientists know that Salk's vaccine was completely effective. Though it happens rarely, Sabin's live-virus vaccine can actually cause polio. So now in the U.S., doctors at the Centers for Disease Control and Prevention in Atlanta, Georgia, recommend vaccinating children only with the killed-virus vaccine.

The current goal is to make polio disappear worldwide by the end of 2000.

How AIDS Changed America

By David Jefferson
Newsweek, May 15, 2006

Jeanne White-Ginder sits at home, assembling a scrapbook about her son, Ryan. She pastes in newspaper stories about his fight to return to the Indiana middle school that barred him in 1985 for having AIDS. She sorts through photos of Ryan with Elton John, Greg Louganis and others who championed his cause. She organizes mementos from his PBS special, "I Have AIDS: A Teenager's Story." "I just got done with his funeral. Eight pages. That was very hard," says White-Ginder, who buried her 18-year-old son in 1991, seven years after he was diagnosed with the disease, which he contracted through a blood product used to treat hemophiliacs. The scrapbook, along with Ryan's bedroom, the way his mother left it when he died, will be part of an exhibit at the Children's Museum of Indianapolis on three children who changed history: Anne Frank. Ruby Bridges. And Ryan White. "He put a face to the epidemic, so people could care about people with AIDS," his mother says.

At a time when the mere threat of avian flu or SARS can set off a coast-to-coast panic—and prompt the federal government to draw up contingency plans and stockpile medicines—it's hard to imagine that the national response to the emergence of AIDS ranged from indifference to hostility. But that's exactly what happened when gay men in 1981 began dying of a strange array of opportunistic infections.* President Ronald Reagan didn't discuss AIDS in a public forum until a press conference four years into the epidemic, by which time more than 12,000 Americans had already died. (He didn't publicly utter the term "AIDS" until 1987.) People with the disease were routinely evicted from their homes, fired from jobs and denied health insurance. Gays were demonized by the extreme right wing: Reagan adviser Pat Buchanan editorialized in 1983, "The poor homosexuals—they have declared war against nature, and now nature is exacting an awful retribution." In much of the rest of the culture, AIDS was simply treated as the punch line to a tasteless joke: "I just heard the Statue of Liberty has AIDS" Bob Hope quipped during the rededication ceremony of the statue in 1986. "Nobody knows if she got it from the mouth of the Hudson or the Staten Island Fairy." Across the river in Manhattan, a generation of young adults was attending more funerals than weddings.

---

* See Appendix for a timeline on *25 Years of AIDS*.

As AIDS made its death march across the nation, killing more Americans than every conflict from World War II through Iraq, it left an indelible mark on our history and culture. It changed so many things in so many ways, from how the media portray homosexuality to how cancer patients deal with their disease. At the same time, AIDS itself changed, from a disease that killed gay men and drug addicts to a global scourge that has decimated the African continent, cut a large swath through black America and infected almost as many women as men worldwide. The death toll to date: 25 million and counting. Through the crucible of AIDS, America was forced to face its fears and prejudices—fears that denied Ryan White a seat in school for a year and a half, prejudices that had customers boycotting restaurants with gay chefs. "At first, a ton of people said that whoever gets AIDS deserves to have AIDS, deserves to literally suffer all the physical pain that the virus carries with it," says Tom Hanks, who won an Oscar for playing a gay lawyer dying of the disease in 1993's "Philadelphia." "But that didn't hold." Watching a generation of gay men wither and die, the nation came to acknowledge the humanity of a community it had mostly ignored and reviled. "AIDS was the great unifier," says Craig Thompson, executive director of AIDS Project Los Angeles and HIV-positive for 25 years.

> Through the crucible of AIDS, America was forced to face its fears and prejudices.

Without AIDS, and the activism and consciousness-raising that accompanied it, would gay marriage even be up for debate today? Would we be welcoming "Will & Grace" into our living rooms or weeping over "Brokeback Mountain"? Without red ribbons, first worn in 1991 to promote AIDS awareness, would we be donning rubber yellow bracelets to show our support for cancer research? And without the experience of battling AIDS, would scientists have the strategies and technologies to develop the antiviral drugs we'll need to battle microbial killers yet to emerge?

AIDS, of course, did happen. "Don't you dare tell me there's any good news in this," says Larry Kramer, who has been raging against the disease—and those who let it spread unchecked—since it was first identified in 1981. "We should be having a national day of mourning!" True. But as we try to comprehend the carnage, it's impossible not to acknowledge the displays of strength, compassion and, yes, love, that were a direct result of all that pain and loss. Without AIDS, we wouldn't have the degree of patient activism we see today among people with breast cancer, lymphoma, ALS and other life-threatening diseases. It was Kramer, after all, who organized 10,000 frustrated AIDS patients into ACT UP, a street army chanting "Silence equals death" that marched on the White House and shut down Wall Street, demanding more government funding for research and quicker access to drugs that might save lives. "The only thing that makes people fight is fear. That's what we discovered about AIDS activism" Kramer says.

Fear can mobilize, but it can also paralyze—which is what AIDS did when it first appeared. And no one—not the government, not the media, not the gay community itself—reacted fast enough to head off disaster. In the fiscally and socially conservative climate of Reagan's America, politicians were loath to fund research into a new pathogen that was killing mostly gay men and intravenous drug users. "In the first years of AIDS, I imagine we felt like the folks on the rooftops during Katrina, waiting for help," says Dr. Michael Gottlieb, the Los Angeles immunologist credited as the first doctor to recognize the looming epidemic. When epidemiologist Donald Francis of the federal Centers for Disease Control in Atlanta tried to get $30 million in funding for an AIDS-prevention campaign, "it went up to Washington and they said f--- off," says Francis, who quit the CDC soon after, defeated.

"Gay Cancer," as it was referred to at the time, wasn't a story the press wanted to cover—especially since it required a discussion of gay sex. While the media had a field day with Legionnaire's disease, toxic shock syndrome and the Tylenol scare, few outlets paid much attention to the new syndrome, even after scores of people had died. The New York Times ran fewer than a dozen stories about the new killer in 1981 and 1982, almost all of them buried inside the paper. (NEWSWEEK, for that matter, didn't run its first cover story on what "may be the public-health threat of the century" until April 1983.) The Wall Street Journal first reported on the disease only after it had spread to heterosexuals: NEW, OFTEN-FATAL ILLNESS IN HOMOSEXUALS TURNS UP IN WOMEN, HETEROSEXUAL MALES, read the February 1982 headline. Even the gay press missed the story at first: afraid of alarming the community and inflaming antigay forces, editors at the New York Native slapped the headline DISEASE RUMORS LARGELY UNFOUNDED atop the very first press report about the syndrome, which ran May 18, 1981. There were a few notable exceptions, particularly the work of the late Randy Shilts, an openly gay journalist who convinced his editors at the San Francisco Chronicle to let him cover AIDS as a full-time beat: that reporting led to the landmark 1987 book "And the Band Played On," a detailed account of how the nation's failure to take AIDS seriously allowed the disease to spread exponentially in the early '80s.

Many gay men were slow to recognize the time bomb in their midst, even as people around them were being hospitalized with strange, purplish skin cancers and life-threatening pneumonia. Kramer and his friends tried to raise money for research during the 1981 Labor Day weekend in The Pines, a popular gay vacation spot on New York's Fire Island. "When we opened the collection boxes, we could not believe how truly awful the results were," says Kramer. The total? $769.55. "People thought we were a bunch of creeps with our GIVE TO GAY CANCER signs, raining on the parade of Pines' holiday festivities." The denial in some corners of the gay community would continue for years. Many were reluctant to give up the sexual liberation they believed they'd earned: as late as 1984, the community was bitterly debating whether to close San Francisco's gay bathhouses, where men were having unprotected sex with any number of partners in a single night.

With death a constant companion, the gay community sobered up from the party that was the '70s and rose to meet the unprecedented challenge of AIDS. There was no other choice, really: they had been abandoned by the nation, left to fend for themselves. "It's important to remember that there was a time when people did not want to use the same bathroom as a person with AIDS, when cabdrivers didn't want to pick up patients who had the disease, when hospitals put signs on patients' doors that said WARNING. DO NOT ENTER," recalls Marjorie Hill, executive director of Gay Men's Health Crisis in New York. Organizations like GMHC sprang up around the country to provide HIV patients with everything from medical care to counseling to food and housing. "Out of whole cloth, and without experience, we built a healthcare system that was affordable, effective and humane," says Darrel Cummings, chief of staff of the Los Angeles Gay & Lesbian Center. "I can't believe our community did what it did while so many people were dying." Patients took a hands-on approach to managing their disease, learning the intricacies of T-cell counts and grilling their doctors about treatment options. And they shared what they learned with one another. "There's something that a person with a disease can only get from another person with that disease. It's support and information and inspiration," says Sean Strub, who founded the magazine Poz for HIV-positive readers.

It took a movie star to get the rest of the nation's attention. In the summer of 1985, the world learned that Rock Hudson—the romantic leading man who'd been a symbol of American virility—was not only gay, but had full-blown AIDS. "It was a bombshell event," says Gottlieb, who remembers standing on the helipad at UCLA Medical Center, waiting for his celebrity patient to arrive, as news helicopters circled overhead. "For many Americans, it was their first awareness at all of AIDS. This prominent man had been diagnosed, and the image of him looking as sick as he did really stuck." Six years later, basketball legend Magic Johnson announced he was HIV-positive, and the shock waves were even bigger. A straight, healthy-looking superstar athlete had contracted the "gay" disease. "It can happen to anybody, even me, Magic Johnson" the 32-year-old announced to a stunned nation, as he urged Americans to practice safe sex.

Given the tremendous stigma, most well-known public figures with AIDS tried to keep their condition a secret. Actor Brad Davis, the star of "Midnight Express," kept his diagnosis hidden for six years, until he died in 1991. "He assumed, and I think rightly so, that he wouldn't be able to find work," says his widow, Susan Bluestein, a Hollywood casting director. After Davis died, rumors flew that he must have been secretly gay. "That part of the gossip mill was the most hurtful to me and my daughter," says Bluestein, who acknowledges in her book "After Midnight" that her husband was a drug addict and unfaithful—but not gay.

With the disease afflicting so many of their own, celebrities were quick to lend support and raise money. Elizabeth Taylor was among the first, taking her friend Rock Hudson's hand in public, before the TV cameras and the world, to dispel the notion that AIDS was something you could catch through casual contact. Her gesture seems quaint today, but in 1985—when the tabloids were awash with speculation that Hudson could have infected actress Linda Evans by simply kissing her during a love scene in "Dynasty"—Taylor's gesture was revolutionary. She became the celebrity face of the American Foundation for AIDS Research. "I've lost so many friends," Taylor says. "I have so many friends who are HIV-positive and you just wonder how long it's going to be. And it breaks your heart."

If TV was slow to deal with AIDS, cinema was downright glacial.

Behind the scenes, Hollywood wasn't nearly as progressive as it likes to appear. John Erman recalls the uphill battle getting the 1985 AIDS drama, "An Early Frost," on TV. "The meetings we had with NBC's Standards and Practices [the network's censors] were absolutely medieval," says Erman. One of the censors' demands: that the boyfriend of the main character be portrayed as "a bad guy" for infecting him: "They did not want to show a positive gay relationship," Erman recalls. Ultimately, with the support of the late NBC Entertainment president Brandon Tartikoff, Erman got to make the picture he wanted—though major advertisers refused to buy commercial time during the broadcast. Within a decade, AIDS had changed the face of television. In 1991, "thirtysomething" featured a gay character who'd contracted the disease. And in 1994, on MTV's "The Real World," 23-year-old Pedro Zamora, who died later that same year, taught a generation of young people what it meant to be HIV-positive.

If TV was slow to deal with AIDS, cinema was downright glacial. "Longtime Companion," the first feature film about the disease, didn't make it to the screen until 1990, nine years into the epidemic. "There was a lot of talk before the movie came out about how this was going to hurt my career, the same way there was talk about Heath Ledger in 'Brokeback Mountain'," says Bruce Davison, who received an Oscar nomination for his role. As for "Philadelphia," Hanks is the first to admit "it was late to the game."

Broadway was the major exception when it came to taking on AIDS as subject matter—in part because so many early casualties came from the world of theater. "I remember in 1982 sitting in a restaurant with seven friends of mine. All were gay men either working or looking to work in the theater, and we were talking about AIDS," recalls Tom Viola, executive director of Broadway Cares/Equity Fights AIDS. "Of those eight guys, four are dead, and two, including myself, are HIV-positive." By the time Tony Kushner's Pulitzer Prize-winning "Angels in America" made its Broadway debut in 1993, some 60 plays about the disease had opened in New York. Producer Jeffrey Seller remembers how he was told he "could never do a show on Broadway that's about, quote unquote, AIDS, homosexuality and drug addiction." He's talking about "Rent," which a decade later still draws capacity crowds.

The world of "Rent" is something of an artifact now. Just before it hit Broadway in 1996, scientists introduced the anti-retroviral drug cocktails that have gone on to extend the lives of millions of patients with HIV. Since then, the urgency that once surrounded the AIDS fight in the United States has ebbed, as HIV has come to be seen as a chronic, rather than fatal, condition. But the drugs aren't a panacea—despite the fact that many people too young to remember the funerals of the '80s think the new medications have made it safe to be unsafe. "Everywhere I go, I'm meeting young people who've just found out they've been infected, many with drug-resistant strains of the virus," says Cleve Jones, who two decades ago decided to start stitching a quilt to honor a friend who had died of AIDS. That quilt grew to become an iconic patchwork of more than 40,000 panels, each one the size of a grave, handmade by loved ones to honor their dead. Ever-expanding, it was displayed several times in Washington, transforming the National Mall into what Jones had always intended: a colorful cemetery that would force the country to acknowledge the toll of AIDS. "If I'd have known 20 years ago that in 2006 I'd be watching a whole new generation facing this tragedy, I don't think I would have had the strength to continue," says Jones, whose own HIV infection has grown resistant to treatment.

Inner strength is what has allowed people living with HIV to persevere. "They think I'm gonna die. You know what, they better not hold their breath," Ryan White once told his mother. Though given six months to live when he was diagnosed with HIV, Ryan lived five and a half years, long enough to prod a nation into joining the fight against AIDS. When he died in 1990 at the age of 18, Congress named a new comprehensive AIDS funding act after him. But the real tribute to Ryan has been the ongoing efforts of his mother. "I think the hostility around the epidemic is still there. And because of religious and moral issues, it's been really hard to educate people about this disease and be explicit," says White-Ginder, who continues to give speeches about watching her son live and die of AIDS. "We should not still be facing this disease." Sadly, we are.

II. Preventing, Controlling, and Eradicating Epidemic Outbreaks

Editor's Introduction

A quick glance at some recent media predictions would suggest that the Earth is overdue for a pandemic. In our information-saturated modern world, the threat of a particular disease evolving into the next plague is sometimes overhyped, leading many people to conclude that a medical crisis is far more grave than a less hysterical perspective would suggest. In these instances it is easy to imagine a "killer virus"—an apocalyptic outbreak so devastating that millions will be sickened or killed. Sometimes just reading the names of particular diseases causes a collective chill to run down our spines. Indeed, the Ebola virus, SARS, and avian flu, among others, carry with them an implicit sense of dread that far exceeds the number of deaths for which they are responsible. However, there are other instances when the true impact of such diseases is vastly underreported, particularly when their victims reside in the developing world. There *are* epidemics occurring right now, whether or not we in the industrialized world are aware of them. Though we now have the ability to access obscure information in a matter of moments, the suffering of the world's poor too often remains out of sight, especially when it doesn't directly affect our own lives.

Whether hyped or ignored, epidemic diseases are having a profound impact on people throughout the world. Therefore, global efforts are continually under way, through international bodies such as the World Health Organization (WHO), aid groups, and national institutes of health, not only to prevent the spread of disease, but also to find medicines and treatments that will bring about their eradication. Though the medical community is in agreement that something must be done to cure the sick and prevent epidemic deaths, what often goes unmentioned are the vigorous debates going on within the community itself as to how best to address a particular outbreak. Occasionally, these debates spill over into the media. A sampling of these efforts—and their accompanying debates—is presented in this chapter.

Collected in this section are articles that discuss the means by which a number of deadly epidemics can be prevented, controlled, or eradicated. In the first article, "Rules of Contagion," Bob Holmes addresses a number of outbreaks currently challenging the medical community and describes the ways in which they are being combated. In an article for *Industrial Management*, "Disease and Globalization: On a Fast Track," Fariborz Ghadar and Beth Hardy discuss the ways in which a globalized economy is hastening the spread of epidemics. In addition to detailing how diseases are transmitted, as well as their impact on society at large, the authors cite ways governments and corporations can react to outbreaks. They likewise discuss opportunities for "information sharing" that will become available should an outbreak require an international response.

From the *Virginia Quarterly Review*, "The Scourge of AIDS in Africa: And Why We Must Act Now," discusses the lack of interest the West seems to have for AIDS victims in Africa. In "How to Wipe Out AIDS in 45 Years," published in *Maclean's*, Jessica Werb reports on a controversial theory that holds that education is not necessarily the most effective means to fight HIV infection. Instead, Dr. Julio Montaner of Canada's B.C. Centre for Excellence in HIV/AIDS argues that governments should focus on expanding access to anti-retroviral therapy.

In the next article, "Global Plan to Stop Tuberculosis," published in the *UN Chronicle*, the author reports that despite considerable investment in controlling tuberculosis, progress has been irregular at best, particularly in African nations where the political leadership hasn't responded as vigorously as it should. Finally, in an article from *Foreign Policy*, "Polio," Julie L. Gerberding explains how this long-feared disease moves closer to worldwide eradication as more and more people are immunized.

Rules of Contagion

By Bob Holmes
New Scientist, October 28, 2006

France, 1918: a new, lethal strain of influenza sweeps through the trenches, killing even young, fit soldiers. Within weeks the outbreak has spread to ports of call in Africa, North America and onward. Over the next two years, at least 20 million people worldwide will die in the worst epidemic since the black death.

Democratic Republic of Congo, 2002: Ebola virus resurfaces, killing nearly 90 per cent of those who catch it. The epidemic does not spread much beyond the country's borders, however, and within months it fades away, leaving a total death toll of just 128.

Your town, last winter: cold viruses rage through schools and offices. Almost everyone catches at least one, yet the epidemic rarely causes sufferers more than a few days' stuffiness and discomfort.

Three diseases, three widely different outcomes. Why do some pathogens cause deadly pandemics while others result in just a local crisis or widespread but minor inconvenience? It's no trifling question: if we could answer it, we could predict whether newly emerging diseases are likely to explode into an epic plague or fizzle out like a damp squib, and could also spot potentially fatal diseases lurking in the wings. Better yet, knowing how and why some pathogens take the evolutionary road to Armageddon, we might be able to devise ways to alter their destiny, stacking the evolutionary deck in our favour to produce milder diseases.

You'd be forgiven for calling this wishful thinking. It certainly isn't easy to explain why some pathogens turn really nasty. Yet, as specialists gain insight into the way diseases emerge and spread, they are beginning to understand the complex evolutionary pressures that determine just how contagious a particular disease will become, and how much of a wallop it will pack. So what can these insights tell us about the threat posed by the likes of bird flu and SARS? Can they help us identify other possible pandemics, or even avert the next "big one"?

The key feature to worry about in any disease is its level of virulence—that is, how sick it will make you. For many years, the standard view among experts was that pathogens inevitably evolve to be less virulent over time. After all, the reasoning went, any germ that kills its host is out of a home, so a pathogen should prefer its host to be up and about, spreading the infection to others. The nasty diseases, in this view, are either relative newcomers to humans or else accidental colonists from other species that have not yet reached a gentler evolutionary equilibrium.

Take the H5N1 strain of bird flu. It is certainly nasty now, killing around 50 per cent of the people it has infected so far, but that's because it is not yet readily transmissible between humans. If that happens, it will surely become less virulent so that it no longer poses such a serious threat. Right? "I hear this all the time," says Irene Eckstrand, who directs an infectious-disease research programme at the US National Institute of General Medical Sciences in Bethesda, Maryland. "In fact, there's no data to back it up."

What is emerging instead is a more nuanced view of how virulence evolves. In this new understanding, pathogens can evolve widely different levels of virulence depending on their circumstances. The crucial factor seems to be transmission—and in particular the manner and ease of a pathogen's spread. Diseases such as respiratory viruses, which are passed on by sneezing, coughing and other forms of direct contact, depend on an infected person being able to move around and mingle. For these pathogens, you would indeed expect evolution to favour low virulence. Sure enough, diseases spread by direct contact, such as the hundreds of viral infections collectively referred to as the common cold, do tend to be innocuous.

> Diseases such as respiratory viruses . . . depend on an infected person being able to move around and mingle.

At the other extreme, diseases spread by mosquitoes or other vectors have much less to lose by disabling their host. "If a human is feeling a little delirious from malaria, that person will still transmit the malaria as well—even better, since a delirious human is less likely to swat the mosquito," says Paul Ewald, an evolutionary biologist at the University of Louisville in Kentucky, who has been one of the most outspoken proponents of the new view of disease evolution. Again this tallies with reality: vector-borne diseases such as malaria, yellow fever and sleeping sickness are among the world's most virulent infectious diseases. Similarly, water-borne diseases and those spread via faeces are likely to severely sicken their host.

Influenza, which we tend to think of as a respiratory disease, may owe some of its virulence to this principle, since it is transmitted via faecal-oral contact in its native waterfowl hosts. Nevertheless, Ewald is optimistic that the H5N1 strain will become less deadly if it evolves the ability to spread from human to human. In its present form, it targets the delicate cells lining the alveoli, deep within the lungs. To become more contagious, it would have to shift its infection site to somewhere higher up in the lungs to improve its chances of being coughed up in significant numbers. "When it infects the alveoli, you get a lot of damage, you get immune over-response," says Ewald. "When you infect the upper respiratory tract, you don't have that damage. So you should see virulence plummet."

There is another important consideration, though. A pathogen's evolutionary path is also likely to depend on its durability. Those that can survive a long time outside their host—on doorknobs or in bedding, for example—can simply sit and wait for a new host to come to them, rather than depending on their current one to pass them on. In that case, even direct-contact pathogens may pay little price for becoming more virulent.

That's exactly what Ewald and Bruno Walther of the University of Copenhagen in Denmark found when they compared the mortality rate and survival time outside the host for 16 pathogens of the human respiratory tract. The six most deadly, causing smallpox, diphtheria, tuberculosis, influenza, pertussis (whooping cough) and pneumonia, were also able to hang on the longest outside people—up to several weeks or months (*Biological Reviews*, vol 79, p 849).

With this in mind, Ewald says the first thing public health officials should test when they encounter a potential new disease is the pathogen's durability, which should take little more than a week. "If it's not durable, it is not as much of a concern," he says.

By this measure we should not worry too much about Ebola, which does not last long outside its host and so is unlikely to spark a major epidemic, despite its high virulence. High on Ewald's worry list, however, is the highly durable monkeypox virus, a pathogen that presently occurs mostly in central and western Africa in a variety of host animals, including monkeys, rats, mice and rabbits. Monkeypox was first recorded in humans in 1970, and there have been several outbreaks since, including one in the US in 2003 when people come into contact with infected pet prairie dogs. "To me, these are of more concern than outbreaks of Ebola," says Ewald.

Diseases such as SARS and bird flu, which are much more virulent than their durability would predict, do not follow this pattern because they have evolved in other host species and only accidentally infect humans, says Ewald. If and when they make the jump to humans, natural selection should rapidly lower their virulence, he predicts.

Understanding the forces that influence disease evolution does not only highlight potential trouble spots. Ewald also believes it might let us turn evolution to our own end to discourage serious diseases from emerging. The idea is that any public health measures that reduce a pathogen's ability to move from host to host should favour pathogens with lower virulence, since they can improve their odds of spreading to a new host by letting their current one live longer.

Ewald cites an example of this in practice. In the early 1990s, the cholera bacterium *Vibrio cholerae* arrived in Peru from Asia and quickly spread throughout Latin America. Within three years, cholera strains in Chile had evolved to produce less toxin, while in contrast, strains in Ecuador produced more. Ewald puts this down to the fact that Chile's drinking water is generally clean, making it more difficult for cholera to spread from very sick people, whereas the more contaminated water supplies in Ecuador provide an easy transmission route.

In a similar vein, simply mosquito-proofing houses and hospitals in malarial regions should favour the mildest strains of the disease. "If somebody is really sick, they're going to be in bed," says Ewald. "And if they are in a mosquito-proofed dwelling, the mosquitoes aren't going to get to them. They are only going to get to the people that are up and moving around—and those tend to be people with a milder strain."

Further Complications

While Ewald's proposals sound like simple good sense, not everyone is convinced by his arguments about the link between virulence and transmissibility. "They're related, of course, but they're related in very complicated ways that often defy the more simplistic efforts at theorising," says Carl Bergstrom, an evolutionary biologist at the University of Washington in Seattle.

> The apparent virulence of a disease sometimes has more to do with the host than with the pathogen.

For one thing, virulence is sometimes just a by-product of chance events or competition among pathogens within a host, rather than being a long-term evolved response. Jim Bull, an evolutionary geneticist at the University of Texas in Austin, points to polio and meningitis. The pathogens causing both these diseases are common (or at least used to be in the case of polio) and mostly harmless human colonists. They only cause disease on the rare occasions when they invade the central nervous system, which is an evolutionary dead end because pathogens that deep within the body are unlikely to find their way out to a new host.

In addition, the apparent virulence of a disease sometimes has more to do with the host than with the pathogen. Sepsis and meningitis, for example, are dangerous because of our own immune system's excessive reaction to the invaders. "It is the host over-response that leads to virulence. If we didn't over-respond, we would be perfectly okay," says Bruce Levin, a population and evolutionary biologist at Emory University in Atlanta, Georgia. What's more, two new studies indicate that the H5N1 strain of flu does much of its damage in this way, as did the 1918 flu (*Nature Medicine*, DOI: 10.1038/nm1493, and *Nature*, DOI: 10.1038/nature05181).

Even something as simple as variation between individual immune responses to a pathogen can be enough to mess up predictions of how virulence evolves. When Bergstrom and his team used a mathematical model of infection to study this, they found that small differences in immune response made a big difference to a pathogen's final virulence (*Evolution*, vol 56, p 213).

POINT OF NO RETURN

By Bob Holmes

Many of the diseases that concern us most did not start out as human diseases at all. Instead, the pathogens that cause influenza, Ebola, SARS and the like began life in other animals and jumped to people by accident. Such cross-infections happen all the time, but most of them sputter out quietly because the pathogen, adapted to its usual host, reproduces poorly in humans or lacks an easy way to get from one person to the next—in short, it is not very contagious. The successful human diseases are the ones that do something about that.

In theory, at least, as long as every person who catches a disease gets it from the original host species, the pathogen's success in that original host will be what drives its evolution, and natural selection will keep it fine-tuned for that species. As soon as a pathogen begins to spread directly from person to person, however, the evolutionary landscape suddenly changes, and the heavy artillery of microbial evolution can be brought to bear on adapting to the new host: us.

This happens when each infected person, on average, passes the disease along to one other person. Pathogens approaching this threshold, although not yet adapted to a human host, have the greatest chance of stringing together a series of person-to-person infections by pure happenstance. That lucky run could give a virus enough time to evolve specific human adaptations, according to mathematical models by Carl Bergstrom from the University of Washington in Seattle and his colleagues (NATURE, vol 426, p 658).

This threshold is a key battlefront in the fight to keep new diseases from jumping to humans. "Even modest gains in reducing the probability of human-to-human transmission can greatly reduce the probability of the virus evolving enough to become an effective pathogen," says Bergstrom. Fortunately, common-sense precautions such as good sanitation and minimising contact with infected people go a long way toward this end already. "When we try to protect healthcare workers from catching bird flu, we are not only looking after them. We're taking a crucial step in reducing the chance that bird flu will emerge as an important human pathogen," says Bergstrom.

There is one other step we can take to reduce the risk of new diseases emerging—one that has been largely ignored of late. Knowing your enemy means careful surveillance of viruses in the wild to compile a rogue's gallery of likely offenders. "There's hardly anyone looking for viruses any more," says Scott Weaver from the University of Texas Medical Branch in Galveston. "We're not even prepared to know what has the potential to emerge out there."

"This was one of many things we came across that left me feeling that virulence evolution may not have these big, beautiful, simplistic, powerful laws when applied at the level of organisms with complex immune systems," Bergstrom says. "I'm a theorist, so I hate to admit this, but for this particular problem, it seems like the details matter tremendously."

Such details have convinced some experts that there is little point in trying to influence the evolution of virulence through measures that affect a disease's transmission. Ewald, however, points out that a pathogen's virulence can sometimes change remarkably quickly. Cholera in Chile is just one example; others include the myxomatosis virus that decimated rabbits in Australia and then evolved into a less lethal form. He does admit, however, that it is unclear whether these are rare exceptions or the norm. "We really need some experiments here," Ewald says.

For instance, he suggests that development agencies that know they can only afford to install clean drinking water in a certain proportion of villages in an area could do so in a way that would allow epidemiologists to glean some useful information. They could, for example, compare the clean-water villages with the unimproved ones to see whether water-borne diseases have evolved lower virulence in the former. "That, I think, is an ethically acceptable experiment."

Meanwhile, the sorts of measures that public health officials might take to encourage the evolution of reduced virulence can only be to the good. After all, clean water, mosquito netting, even simple measures such as hand-washing and staying at home when ill, are excellent measures to help prevent epidemics in the short term. Any evolutionary benefit would be an added bonus.

Disease and Globalization

On a Fast Track

BY FARIBORZ GHADAR AND BETH HARDY
INDUSTRIAL MANAGEMENT, JANUARY/FEBRUARY 2006

Executive Summary

While epidemics have been around for as long as humanity's existence, their spread was once held in check by geography. However, the proliferation of high-speed global transport of people and livestock has opened the floodgates for disease transmission. Private business must find its role in responding to disease outbreaks.

In this era of globalization, infectious disease thrives along with cross-border integration—including the movement of goods, labor, and transportation. Health and security have become key areas of both business and government observation. The international community already contends with viruses such as HIV, malaria, SARS, and tuberculosis. As the world becomes more integrated, companies, governments, and individuals are faced with the challenges and opportunities that disease presents.

Epidemics take their tolls on societies in a variety of ways: loss of life, political instability, and economic stagnation accompany epidemics sweeping the world today. In the face of these health crises, governments and corporations must respond quickly and effectively or risk losing citizens, workers, and consumers.

How Epidemics Begin and Spread

Epidemics and the diseases that cause them are not new. Diseases have decimated the populations of every continent. In the 1300s, the bubonic plague, or Black Death as it was commonly known, swept through Europe, killing up to 30 percent of the population. Arriving in 1346, most likely due to new trade patterns and army movements, the plague moved quickly through Europe over the next four years.

The plague was a factor, at least in part, for altering the makeup of society. The massive loss of workers caused the demise of the feudal system, and the Renaissance was born.

This story of epidemic and economic recovery is repeated over and over in the history of humanity. Business leaders must recognize the awesome impact disease can have on a stable world. The ruling class of the Middle Ages did not take into account the possibility of a disease drastically altering the fabric of their society. Today's business leaders can learn from that mistake. Europeans did not track the movement of the plague; they were unaware that trade was facilitating the development of the disease.

Now, technology enables epidemiologists to study the movement of disease almost to the person. More is known about transmission modes, incubation periods, and the contagious nature of diseases. The World Health Organization and many governments have come together to monitor, track, and prevent epidemics before they reach the level of the Black Death.

However, with new technology comes a new challenge. We must contend with the speed at which people and goods move around the planet. Planes, boats, high-speed trains, trucks, cars, and every other type of transportation can move anything anywhere at breakneck speed. This means that diseases no longer take years to reach new geographic areas. Pathogens can arrive within hours. Travelers, business people, tourists, diplomats, and reporters become innocent transporters of deadly diseases.

> As populations continue to interconnect, the likelihood of epidemics and pandemics of infectious disease increases.

As populations continue to interconnect, the likelihood of epidemics and pandemics of infectious disease increases. Compared to the plague, which took four years to spread, SARS originated in China and spread rapidly to 30 countries within weeks, with relatively severe outbreaks in Toronto, Taiwan, and Beijing. As global health organizations struggled to identify and contain the virus, SARS grounded airlines, hurt businesses, and even caused riots in China.

Because trade and travel now link so many societies, SARS-like epidemics and their human and economic consequences can no longer come as a surprise. Businesses must be able to adapt quickly to changed market conditions brought about by such epidemics.

The stakes associated with this tectonic force are high. Infectious diseases kill millions of people every year and, as the SARS virus demonstrated, can quickly generate economic turmoil on a global scale. The global economic impact of SARS was estimated at $30 billion, with an estimated $12.3 billion in losses in Asia alone.

Countries need a global health infrastructure that responds quickly and effectively to epidemics such as the avian flu, SARS, or terrorist-induced disease outbreaks. In this era of increased economic and social integration, an outbreak in one country can develop into a global pandemic in a matter of days. As a result, governments, non-government organizations, and private companies must devise health care solutions that cross borders as effectively as the infectious agents they work to contain.

Disease and Society

Infectious disease significantly affects economic growth and development, especially in countries with high disease burdens. In many developing countries, HIV/AIDS has decimated the labor force and overwhelmed already struggling education and health care systems. The catastrophic effects will burden those countries for generations to come.

While the world struggles to prevent new outbreaks, current diseases continue to spread. AIDS, tuberculosis, and malaria kill approximately 6 million people a year, which is about 16,000 people a day. The spread of these preventable diseases takes its toll on the countries where they occur and generally correlate to a low level of public health and a high level of poverty. Governments must contend with these two problems in their efforts to stop infectious disease.

It is important to note that those countries with the most underdeveloped public health services record the highest infection rates. Of the 42 million people now diagnosed with AIDS worldwide, for example, 95 percent live in the developing world—with Africa and India reporting the majority of new cases.

Pre-emptive spending on diseases should prove beneficial to businesses, offering the twofold benefits of making money on infrastructure efforts and saving money by diverting problems. Businesses should encourage governments to build disease prevention infrastructure.

Local Diseases Are Now Global

Because people now move freely about the planet, we must prepare ourselves for diseases to which our bodies have not developed immunity. It is not just humans who relocate: Diseases invariably tag along.

As current epidemics are fought, new ones arise daily. It is feared that the next SARS-like outbreak is already underway in the form of avian flu. Dozens of people have already died from the avian flu virus (H5N1), which continues to be discovered in new countries. The World Health Organization and America's Center for Disease Control and Prevention are now becoming concerned about a flu pandemic like the 1918 outbreak in Spain that killed more than 20 million people. Given travel and urban overcrowding, the disease is unlikely to stay in one country or area should an outbreak occur. Billions of dollars have been earmarked by the United States to combat an Asian disease that has killed two dozen people halfway around the world. This is but one of many steps the world needs to take to fight against current and developing diseases.

Before indigenous diseases move to new and unconquered lands, the best treatment is still often local. Frequently, it is the local medical community that is the most adept at identifying and treating something they are familiar with.

This need for local knowledge in non-local places is crucial in the fight against disease. As the United States government has realized this, so must businesses.

Northrop Grumman Information Technology is one of at least eight companies and academic institutions that have been contracted by the United States National Institute of Allergy and Infectious Disease (part of the National Institutes of Health) to compile a database of six known pathogens.

These six pathogens will become part of a centralized, consolidated information set for scientific researchers. Because the bulk of information is being created at research institutions, it is difficult to avoid data replication, a costly and unnecessary process. The goal is for this database to eliminate that problem as well as make local knowledge accessible to the global community

Current plans are that the database will be designed such that additional pathogens can be added. Current costs for the task, all of which are being paid by the U.S. federal government, are estimated at upwards of $83 million. Jobs similar to this one are sure to emerge at a rapid pace as more governments, non-government organizations, and international members of civil society follow the lead of the United States.

Epidemics

In sub-Saharan Africa, 25 million to 28 million people live with AIDS. By 2010, this region will no longer rank as the most HIV-infected region: China, Ethiopia, India, Nigeria, and Russia will become the new centers of the AIDS epidemic. Cumulatively, these states are trying to support between 14 million and 23 million people living with AIDS, numbers that will increase to 75 million people by 2010. These infection rates will reduce productivity, gross domestic product, and foreign direct investment. Today, the AIDS epidemic rages in many developing countries that must also contend with malaria, yellow fever, and dengue fever. Together, these diseases have already orphaned millions of children, discouraged foreign investment, and impaired the healthcare infrastructure.

Government Response

Chinese leaders are taking steps to fight the rising HIV/AIDS epidemic that experts predict in their country. President Hu Jintao and former President Jiang Zemin met with former U.S. President Clinton in New York recently to discuss means for stopping AIDS. China is the only country with 1 billion people, and half of them have never heard of AIDS. The Chinese government is hoping to prevent the spread of HIV/AIDS before it develops into the epidemic proportions already seen in other parts of the world.

The threat of infectious disease in a tightly connected international system is prompting greater cooperation and communication on issues previously deemed too sensitive to report or discuss.

Corporate Response

Hank McKinnell of Pfizer was the only drug company CEO to attend the International AIDS Conference during the summer of 2004 in Bangkok, Thailand. Often criticized for high-priced drugs and opposition to generic knockoffs, Pfizer is addressing the AIDS epidemic as more than an opportunity to donate free medication. However, McKinnell contends that for Pfizer to continue its research and donations to the Third World, developed countries must continue to pay market prices for drugs.

Pfizer is helping build the necessary infrastructure to fight against infectious diseases. In the face of an epidemic such as AIDS, which often times feels too large to control (or for that matter, understand), the steps being taken are extraordinary. On Oct. 20, 2005, the Infectious Diseases Institute was opened in Uganda as a result of the remarkable coming together of The Pfizer Foundation,

---

Threats of bioterrorism and contamination of food and water supplies haunt global leaders and the public.

Makerere University in Uganda, Pangaea Global AIDS Foundation, the Academic Alliance Foundation for AIDS Care and Prevention in Africa, and the Infectious Diseases Society of America. The IDI hopes to treat 300 patients a day and 10,000 patients a year, putting as many as needed on antiretroviral drugs.

IDI also plans to train 250 AIDS specialists a year who will be able to work in rural conditions and train others. Merle Sande of the Academic Alliance Foundation summarized the program as follows: "The IDI reflects true partnerships between academicians in North America and Africa and the public-private sectors who have come together to build infrastructure to combat the most threatening disease to attack mankind."

Terrorism

As the global community contends with naturally created disease, there are those attempting to harness the power of epidemics for destructive purposes. Threats of bioterrorism and contamination of food and water supplies haunt global leaders and the public.

Smallpox is a case in point. Because many countries stopped their smallpox vaccination programs in the 1970s, a biological attack with this potential terrorist weapon would create a humanitarian disaster. In light of this threat, Israel and the United States recently vaccinated their military personnel. Following the Sept. 11 terrorist attacks and the subsequent release of anthrax through the United States postal system, many countries now work to prevent terrorist groups from gaining access to dangerous bio-agents. Infectious disease has become an issue of national and international security for the entire global community.

The fight against bioterrorism is going to be a more different war than has ever been fought before: one to be fought at the cellular level. This cellular-level fight will be a battle of information and containment; this is where business can play a role.

Opportunity, Disease, and Change

What should businesses be doing to prepare for contingencies arising from natural or deliberate epidemics and disease-related volatility? First, they need to engage in scenario-analysis to begin to define their reactions in the event of an epidemic. Second, they should assess the extent to which international and national institutions are prepared for such contingencies—especially because public-private sector partnership is critical to defining and implementing solutions. Third, the growing threat of bioterrorism suggests new possibilities for the private sector to marshal its resources and technological innovation in support of new biodefenses and procedures.

Traditional medical research takes place at one laboratory with one team taking credit for patents and discoveries. Information is kept private while the proprietary information can be published.

By contrast, the Myelin Repair Foundation was started by Scott Johnson, a Silicon Valley executive who was diagnosed with the degenerative disease myelin at the age of 20. Johnson distributes money only to researchers who agree to share their findings without waiting for publication or patents.

For years, foundations have been pumping money into research at various locations, often finding themselves frustrated with the pace of development. The new collaborative method is revolutionizing the medical field as it cuts years off development time. The five labs working for Johnson's foundation believe they have already saved 10 to 15 years on their goal of identifying a drug target and finding a promising compound by 2009.

There are concerns with this new method. Some scientists like the notoriety that accompanies innovation. Others might be driven out of the collaborative teams by intellectual property rights desires. Forcing scientists to share information takes away patenting from one laboratory, which often needs the money from sales of that patent to continue its work. The future of this method is yet to be determined, but for now, there are opportunities for business to play a role.

International disease control will present vast opportunities and challenges to businesses operating in afflicted countries or working to provide containment products and services. The ability of these corporations, along with governments and non-government organizations, to react and respond to outbreaks and to devise solutions that meet the health care needs of the world's population, will be critical to continued global prosperity.

TERMINOLOGY

An epidemic is a sudden severe outbreak of disease within a region or group. A pandemic occurs when an epidemic becomes widespread, affecting a whole region, a continent, or the entire world.

Source: MedicineNet.com

LOCAL DISEASE, GLOBAL IMPLICATION

"Despite some alarming trends, the infectious disease situation . . . is largely encouraging, sometimes in ways that suggest a fundamental change for the better in the landscape of public health. The world is on guard as never before. The threat posed by infectious disease is now perceived to be universally relevant, as the speed and volume of international travel have made an outbreak or epidemic anywhere in the world a potential threat everywhere else. Moreover, the ability of infectious diseases to destabilize societies, so alarmingly demonstrated by AIDS, has brought home the message that local infectious disease problems can have global security implications."

—World Health Organization

WHOSE PROBLEM IS IT?

In a World Economic Forum survey of 8,000 companies, 47 percent of firms believe that AIDS is having or will have an impact on their business. Only 3 percent of the same companies polled were satisfied with their company's response to date. Many companies still cling to the belief that AIDS is not their problem.

Source: The Global Business Coalition on HIV/AIDS.

HELP FROM BUSINESS

"Business brings with it qualities that can turn the tide of the epidemic. The entrepreneurial spirit and problem-solving expertise that the private sector brings to the table means that most companies operate with a core set of skills that can be leveraged to positively impact the epidemic. Efficiency of operations, overcoming obstacles, responsibility for achieving concrete outcomes, and accurately gauging perceptions and human behavior help business to thrive and are prerequisites for success in battling the pandemic locally, nationally, and internationally."

—World Health Organization

GREATER GLOBAL RISK LEADING TO GREATER COLLABORATION

A new trend in funded research is arising, pushed forward by such power players as the Juvenile Diabetes Research Foundation, the Michael J. Fox Foundation for Parkinson's Research, and the newly founded Myelin Repair Foundation for multiple sclerosis research. This trend is one of information sharing as opposed to the age-old information hiding.

The Scourge of AIDS in Africa

And Why We Must Act Now

The Virginia Quarterly Review, Winter 2006

In August 2001, I was strapped into the passenger seat, speeding along the highway between Johannesburg and Pretoria, the capital of South Africa. On the edge of every shantytown and encampment, we passed two invariable landmarks: shacks with men selling stacks of tires and large billboards with slogans like "Condoms make it safer" and "Be wise, condomise." I asked Naas, our guide and driver, about the tires. "Patched and retread from blowouts," he explained. "For the taxis." The taxis were really minivans, crowded tight, mostly with women, headed for service jobs in either of the two cities. Their drivers cover hundreds of miles each day—always speeding, always on treads worn so thin that they are in constant danger of high-speed blowouts.

It's hard not to read such things as emblematic of larger ills in Africa. The entire continent is threadbare, hurtling forward, and constantly on the brink of catastrophe. Of course, that brink is frequently breached—whether by genocide, as in Sudan, or by natural disaster, such as the recent drought in Niger. Americans have always been vaguely aware of such problems and always made good-faith, if misguided, efforts to help. I remember too well plinking away on a cheap Casio keyboard, while the chorus of my classmates earnestly belted out "We Are the World" in the bleak auditorium of my middle school in Pittsburgh, all in an effort to raise money for the starving in Ethiopia. That was 1985, when we still thought such things—Band-Aid, Live Aid—were all it would take to save Africa.

Then came the era of AIDS—an era shrouded in the silence of our government's unwillingness to discuss publicly a sexually transmitted disease, an era clouded by our own lack of moral clarity toward peoples of different races and different cultures with different sexual mores. Were that not enough, in 2000, within a month of my return to the United States, everything changed—as we've grown accustomed to saying. Our well of sympathy for those struggling on foreign soil went dry overnight, and there was little to refill the fount, as rumors swirled first in 2001 that Osama bin Laden had fled to Somalia and later in 2003 that Niger had supplied yellowcake uranium to Saddam Hussein. Though neither claim proved true, we now live in times where the shadow of doubt stretches wider and lingers longer than ever before.

To say we have forgotten the problems of Africa in the last four years would be an understatement. Our government has suspended many of the programs that allow for resettlement of political refugees. We have turned away from enforcing UN demands on African dictators. Worst of all, the Bush administration has made promises for political gain, then broken them for political expediency. In March 2002, for example, President Bush proposed the Millennium Challenge Account, a program by which the United States would increase aid by 50% over the next three years, resulting in an annual increase of $5 billion by fiscal year 2006. Yet, in January 2005, as FY06 approached, Bush requested only $3 billion to fund Millennium Challenge, and Congress cut that amount to $1.75 billion without a struggle from the White House—leaving barely a third of what was originally promised. Little notice has been paid to this broken promise or what it means for Africa.

Let's be clear. The result of our inaction is not simply that programs for AIDS go "underfunded." We cannot accept such bureaucratic language any longer. The real result of our inaction is that 7,000 people die in Africa every day. Rockstar-turned-activist Bono has rightly taken to describing this number as "two 9/11s per day." The tragedy of September 11, 2001, is in no way to be minimized, but as Jann Turner points out later in this issue, the most painful images of that day were the photographs of people hanging from the burning towers, knowing, as we did, the certainty of their deaths. But why then are we not moved by the deaths of so many in Africa? Should they not be that much more painful to us, knowing that they are avoidable deaths? And they are avoidable. Indeed, with the aid of antiretroviral drugs, people living with HIV and AIDS experience what is known as a "Lazarus effect," where the near-dead rise from their sickbeds like Lazarus risen from the grave to walk again among us. Yet only 3% of the 4 million Africans in immediate need of such drugs have access to them. Many of these drugs cost only a dollar a day, but most Africans can't afford this. For less than $1.5 billion annually, we could supply antiretrovirals to the entire continent.

However, it is not merely a matter of treating those already HIV-positive; it is also important to stop the spread of the disease. UNICEF, which recently launched its campaign "Unite for Children, Unite Against AIDS" estimates that 1,400 children die of AIDS-related illnesses every day, but even more alarmingly an additional 1,800 children under the age of fifteen become newly HIV-positive in that same twenty-four hour period. Of these, the Africa aid organization DATA (Debt, AIDS, Trade, Africa) estimates that 1,400 are infected during childbirth. According to AVERT, an international AIDS charity, inexpensive drugs are already available that reduce the chances of a mother transmitting HIV to her child during birth from 40% to 2%—but the United States does not currently fund aid for these medications. As a result, in the next twelve months alone, nearly half a million children, who could have been born healthy, instead will be born HIV-positive in Africa. Most will not live to adulthood. Any way you look at it, millions of children will die from an avoidable infection and a treatable disease.

There is a lot of talk in the halls of Washington these days about morality, about reestablishing America's moral authority, about returning to our country's Christian values. How can any moral American—much less any self-proclaimed Christian—turn away from this challenge? These are the poor. These are the meek, who shall inherit the earth. Before we rush to hang the Ten Commandments in every courthouse, let us first enshrine in our hearts and minds the wisdom of the historical Jesus as set forth in the Beatitudes and the Sermon on the Mount. One need not be churchgoing to share reverence for such teachings. For once in this country, let us remember that the first shall be last, and the last shall be first.

But, if our consciences are not enough, can we at least act in our own enlightened self-interest? Who do we imagine the millions of AIDS orphans, those who avoid infection, will grow up to be? If, as it appears, al Quaeda has gained a foothold in eastern Africa—Somalia, Kenya, Ethiopia, Rwanda, Sudan—then we must do everything in our power to show America's right, and not only its might. If we fail to act now, if we fail to show our compassion, then Africa could easily lapse into the same extremism that consumes the Middle East. If we really mean to make our world safer, then we must work to make allies of our potential enemies. We must befriend now or defend later. This is the choice we face—and what a luxury we enjoy to have such options before us.

Africa has no such choices. The vast majority of the continent shares a common fate without any say in their future. Like those crowded minivans, rushing from the countryside toward Pretoria and Johannesburg, they are merely passengers at the mercy of an unknown driver. I think of them—and the fate of their nation and continent—every time I recall passing yet another tire stand, piled high with repaired radials and whitewalls.

"Are they safe to drive on?" I asked Naas, who answered instead with his own question, "Would you drive on them?"

How to Wipe Out AIDS in 45 Years

By Jessica Werb
Maclean's, August 14–21, 2006

Dr. Julio Montaner, the Argentinian-born director of the internationally acclaimed B.C. Centre for Excellence in HIV/AIDS and president-elect of the International AIDS Society, doesn't exactly think small. On Aug. 4, *The Lancet* published a paper in which Montaner and his colleagues outline a theory to eradicate the global spread of HIV within 4½ decades. And it has nothing to do with condoms, abstinence or free needle exchanges.

The Lancet paper, ambitiously entitled "The case for expanding access to highly active anti-retroviral therapy [HAART] to curb the growth of the HIV epidemic," contends that HAART—which suppresses the number of copies of a virus in an infected individual—is responsible for the reduction and stabilization of HIV infection rates in the developed world, and that aggressively expanding its use could effectively halt the spread of the virus in its tracks. Furthermore, Montaner maintains that implementing such a strategy, which he acknowledges would cost in the hundreds of billions of dollars, is not only good health policy but cost-effective as well.

"We know that in various settings—whether it's in the health care worker exposure setting or the mother-to-child transmission setting, or the sexually active discordant couples where one is HIV-positive and one is not—in any of those settings, the higher the virus load in the infected person, the higher the chances that the other member of the team . . . is going to become infected," he explains.

A few isolated studies, he says, have indicated that infected individuals treated with HAART are much less likely—even "very unlikely"—to transmit the virus. He cites a 2004 ecological study in Taiwan that showed a 53 per cent reduction in new HIV infections after the introduction of free access to HAART; he also notes that in British Columbia, new HIV infections fell from 1995 to 1998 by close to 50 per cent after the introduction of HAART, and have remained stable since. These decreases in infection rates cannot be attributed to changes in sexual behaviour, he says, because while HIV rates were dropping, syphilis rates were increasing in both Taiwan and B.C. In fact, B.C. has been experiencing a syphilis epidemic since the mid-'90s, particularly among gay men. "This suggests that it's not behaviour that is driving this stable, lower rate of HIV infection," says Montaner.

Montaner estimates that approximately 43,000 cases of HIV infection in North America were averted in 2005 due to HAART; this translates to a savings of US$10.3 billion, based on an estimated lifetime treatment cost of US$241,000 per person. Extrapolating on a global scale, Montaner says that if every single HIV-infected individual was given therapy, the prevalence of HIV could be reduced from more than seven cases per 1,000 to 0.1 case per 1,000 in 45 years. The price for such an endeavour? A staggering US$338 billion over 45 years, based on a cost of $365 for generic HAART drugs per person per year.

Montaner is unperturbed by the figures. "Although this would entail a significant expenditure upfront because you will be treating 40 million people in the world as opposed to four million, the curve of expenditures for the 40 million will drop steadily, so that in a decade or two you actually break even, and after that you're laughing all the way to the bank," he says.

His theory begs a number of questions, not least of which is how to deliver treatment on such a massive scale, and how to identify those who require it. And, of course, there's the small matter of who'll be footing the bill. Montaner, ever the idealist, has answers for all of these. The use of rapid HIV tests—one, produced by Vancouver-based bioLytical Laboratories, gained approval from Health Canada in November for point-of-care use and provides results in 60 seconds—would enable health care workers to go into communities and implement mass-scale HIV testing to pinpoint infected individuals. Rapid advances in drugs, like the three-in-one Atripla combination pill that received FDA approval in July (Health Canada is expected to follow shortly) would make adherence to drug regimens much easier.

As for the bill? "If you think about economics, you develop a product for a given market and you do your calculations," says Montaner. "You could say [to drug companies], 'Look, I'm going to protect your profits. You generated this drug with a profit that was based on the North American market or European market or whatever. You know what? We'll give you full profit for that. On top of that, we're going to give you a premium so that you can make drugs for free to distribute to the rest of the world.'" He adds: "If marketing pressures can allow you to get a can of Coke in every corner of the world, that proves that distribution chains are not, should not, and cannot be an impediment to doing what is right."

As to be expected, not everyone is greeting Montaner's theory with enthusiasm. Louise Binder, chair of the Canadian Treatment Action Council, says bluntly, "I'm not buying it. I know about the work that says that people on antiviral therapies tend to have lower viral load in the body. That's all very nice. But [Montaner] wants to use drugs for prevention instead of developing good prevention campaigns. I do not see this in any way being a sensible solution to solving the problem of HIV transmission." She adds: "I think it's got ethical

problems, informed consent problems and cost-containment problems. Treatment itself is toxic. Are you going to put people on treatment who don't need to be there? It's kind of crazy."

She's also concerned about the development of drug-resistant HIV
strains. "There are other, better ways to resolve the problem of HIV
infection than filling everyone we know with the disease full of
drugs to get the viral load down," she insists.

In a statement from the Public Health Agency of Canada, spokesman Alain Desroches echoes Binder's reservations. "The HIV virus
can still be transmitted when on treatment," he says. "This transmission is demonstrated by the detection of mutations associated
with drug resistance among newly diagnosed, untreated individuals. . . . Therefore, in addition to the availability of HAART, any
strategy aimed at significantly reducing HIV transmission needs to
also promote prevention messages and access to HIV testing and
risk-reduction counselling."

"There are other, better ways to resolve the
problem of HIV infection than filling everyone we
know with the disease full of drugs to get the viral
*load down."—***Louise Binder, chair of the Canadian***
Treatment Action Council

Montaner maintains that he sees the expansion of HAART treatment taking place in conjunction with current prevention programs,
and he does not advocate testing or treating patients against their
will. As for resistance, he says studies have shown that while drug
resistance does occur, it does not do so at rates that are any cause
for concern.

Mark Wainberg is director of the McGill AIDS Centre, former
president of the International AIDS Society and chairman of the
organizing committee for the XVI International AIDS Conference
taking place the week of Aug. 13 in Toronto, where Montaner will be
making a plenary address outlining his work. Unlike Binder, he
hails Montaner's work as a significant breakthrough. "I think it's
wonderful, and I think it makes a lot of sense," he says. "We've been
telling people to use condoms for 20 years. Just telling people to use
condoms is not enough of an answer." What makes Montaner's argument so compelling, he says, is its economic component. "It's the
first time someone has done this kind of modelling and cost analysis."

Montaner is ready to test his theory. He's in discussions with the
B.C. Health Ministry and coastal health authorities to develop a
pilot program in B.C. The program would use rapid HIV tests to
aggressively seek out infected individuals and employ an incentive
program to ensure adherence to a drug regimen. Incentives—including, possibly, cash or food—could be given to patients who fully par-

ticipate in treatment programs, comply with drug treatment or achieve predetermined viral load counts. If he does indeed prove that expanded HAART treatment curbs HIV transmission, Montaner says the world will have a bigger problem on its hands than the current epidemic: "It's not that we have HIV, it's that we now know how to handle it. And it's up to the world to decide whether or not we're going to put the effort in to do what needs to be done."

Global Plan to Stop Tuberculosis

Investment in TB Control Works but Progress Uneven

UN Chronicle, March/May 2006

Three of the world's six regions are expected to achieve targets for tuberculosis (TB) control, according to a World Health Organization (WHO) report published on 22 March 2006.

The Americas, South-East Asia and the Western Pacific regions should reach targets set by the World Health Assembly to detect 70 per cent of TB cases and successfully treat 85 per cent of these cases by the end of 2005, according to the *Global Tuberculosis Control 2006*. The report confirms that 26 countries had already met the targets a year ahead of time, two of them being the high-TB burden countries of the Philippines and Viet Nam. It also indicates that five other high-burden countries—Cambodia, China, India, Indonesia and Myamnar—should have reached the targets within the 2005 time frame, though final confirmation will come at the end of 2006.

WHO Director-General Dr. Lee Jong-wook said: "There is clear evidence that investment in TB control works. Even in low-income countries with enormous financial constraints, programmes are operating effectively and producing results. This same commitment needs to be replicated in African countries and other areas where funding and priority for TB control remains fragile."

The latest estimates in the report suggest that 1.7 million people died from TB in 2004 and there were also 8.9 million new cases, with its number per capita rising at 1 per cent per year globally as a consequence of the TB crisis in Africa—a crisis attributed partly to the complications of HIV infection and poor health systems. Eastern Europe, with its high prevalence of multi-drug-resistant tuberculosis (MDR-TB), also continues to have an adverse impact on the global treatment success rates.

Despite the cost-effectiveness of TB control, there is concern that African leaders are still failing to seriously invest in it. Response to the 2005 TB emergency declaration in Africa has been, for the most part, far too sluggish. The report highlights the need for a much more rapid and vigorous response to the African TB emergency, including more ambitious plans that are backed up by more funding from Governments and donors. Kenya is one country that is responding to the emergency declaration's call for "urgent and extraordinary actions" to address TB and TB/HIV. Its Minister of Health, Charity Kaluki Ngilu, said: "Kenya is determined to make a difference. We are taking a strong and decisive lead in TB control through our own national TB emergency plan. This is a strategic plan that lays out the actions and resources required to reduce the misery caused by unnecessary TB deaths."

Other new initiatives, with the shared aim of improving access to TB treatments for all, were also launched in Geneva prior to World TB Day which is 24 March. A set of *International Standards for Tuberculosis Care*, describing the level of care all health practitioners should follow, together with a new *Patients' Charter for Tuberculosis Care*, outlining for the first time the rights and responsibilities of people with TB, were also released on 22 March. The two documents are important inclusions in a new six-point Stop TB Strategy developed by WHO and are highlighted in the Stop TB Partnership's Global Plan to Stop TB, 2006–2015, which was launched in January 2006.

The six components of the new Stop TB Strategy are: pursue high-quality DOTS expansion and enhancement; address TB/HIV, MDR-TB and other challenges; contribute to strengthening the health system; engage all care providers; empower the communities and people with TB; and enable and promote research. The increased momentum around TB control has been stimulated by commitments to the Global Plan to Stop TB, underpinned by the Strategy. However, for the Plan to succeed in saving 14 million extra lives, a ten-year funding gap of $31 billion must be bridged. This is equivalent to just $2 a year from every person in the industrialized world.

Polio

By Julie L. Gerberding
Foreign Policy, September/October 2005

Few causes merit greater celebration than the end of a disease. But despite the dedicated efforts of the last century, the world has only held such a celebration once—when smallpox was eradicated in 1977. Current generations who know smallpox only as a fading scar on the upper arm forget the impact that this global killer had over centuries. Its eradication in the United States alone has saved countless lives and at least $17 billion.

Today, the world is poised to add another disease to the list of those that will no longer threaten humans: polio. As difficult as smallpox eradication was, polio has presented an even tougher challenge. Some polio infections alert doctors with tell-tale paralysis, but for each of these cases, about 200 people may have only minor flu-like symptoms and can silently transmit the disease for weeks. As a logistical challenge, one observer has written, the difference between smallpox and polio eradication is "the difference between extinguishing a candle flame and putting out a forest fire."

Yet we have never been closer to ending the disease. In 1988, there were an estimated 350,000 cases of polio worldwide. In 2005, the confirmed caseload has been slashed to just 760 people in 13 countries. Through national and international leadership, local heroism, and economic investments, immunization rates are climbing in most countries. In 2003, 415 million children in 55 countries were immunized during National Immunization Days, using more than 2.2 billion doses of oral polio vaccine. Most national health services have responded quickly to outbreaks. China, for example, stamped out a potential flare-up last year. The World Health Organization launched a massive preemptive vaccination campaign in Somalia to prevent an outbreak from spreading into the country from neighboring epidemic areas.

The obstacles now are not a lack of vision or inadequate technology; they are civil war and cultural mistrust. Several Nigerian states have, at times, blocked polio immunization campaigns, believing the vaccine to be a Western plot designed to render their women infertile. The August 2003 refusal by the state of Kano resulted in hundreds of children being paralyzed and the virus spreading to neighboring countries. Despite these setbacks, the U.S. Centers for Disease Control and Prevention and its partners around the world believe that polio eradication is within our grasp.

Each global infectious disease poses unique challenges, but the strategy is clear: eradication in one region after another; isolation to a limited number of countries; and aggressive campaigns to break the chain of transmission and infection. In the Americas, public health authorities have already eradicated measles and are stopping the transmission of rubella. We are optimistic that these diseases, and others, will soon go from endangered to extinct. These eradications will be triumphs for public health scientists and practitioners. Even more important, they will be a testament to the power of global cooperation against diseases that recognize no boundaries.

III. Is Avian Flu the Next Epidemic?

Editor's Introduction

As has been widely reported, a strain of avian influenza, the influenza A virus subtype H5N1, also known as the bird flu, has raised great concern among health officials around the world. Since its first appearance in the early days of the 21st century, the bird flu has become endemic in avian populations throughout Southeast Asia, requiring the culling of tens of millions of chickens and other poultry to prevent its spread. Despite these efforts the disease has infected wild-bird populations and has also sickened or killed some people who have come in contact with tainted poultry. However, unlike the Spanish Flu of 1918–19, this strain of influenza is still a specifically avian variety and cannot yet pass easily from person to person or infect humans as an airborne pathogen. Still, the fear of H5N1 mutating into a virus that could effortlessly pass to people has galvanized the world community. One particular cause for worry is the mortality rate: 60 percent of the men and women who were infected with the virus died as a result. General alarms were raised in 2003 when the prominent virologist Robert Webster published an article in *American Scientist* arguing that the world is overdue for the kind of pandemic a mutated variant of H5N1 could provide. In October 2005 David Nabarro, the senior United Nations system coordinator for avian and human influenza, predicted that an outbreak of avian flu in the human population could kill between five million and 150 million people worldwide. Although H5N1 has killed in total about 170 people as of early 2007, health officials across the globe are taking the continued threat seriously and are coordinating their efforts to develop a viable vaccine.

This section of the book is devoted to the efforts the world community is making to combat the next epidemic, which many anticipate will be an outbreak of the avian flu in the human population. In the first selection, "In the Shadow of Pandemic," Tyler A. Kokjohn and Kimbal E. Cooper present a comprehensive overview of the bird flu's history and the preparations being made to combat it, should it start to infect people. Though most agree that the bird flu poses a real threat to humanity, some skeptics remain. In the second article, "Panic Attack," William Speed Weed asks whether the dire predictions of pandemic outbreak are justified by the underlying facts. In the subsequent entry, "What the President Should Have Said About Bird Flu," Nick Schulz describes the criticisms generated by President George W. Bush and the federal government's avian flu preparations. In "Spreading Its Wings," published in *U.S. News & World Report*, Nancy Shute discusses the bird-flu virus and reports on how American health officials are tracking the migration of wild birds, in the hopes of catching a stateside avian flu outbreak early. The final article in this section, "Immediate Treatment Needed for Bird Flu Cases,

Study Says," by Donald G. McNeil Jr., notes that a new report finds that avian flu possesses some of the same characteristics as the Spanish Flu and that those infected would require immediate treatment in order to save their lives.

In the Shadow of Pandemic

By Tyler A. Kokjohn and Kimbal E. Cooper
The Futurist, September/October 2006

A new form of avian influenza ("bird flu") virus is now spreading across the globe and is anticipated to arrive in the Western Hemisphere soon. Although avian influenza is limited primarily to birds, the fact that this flu is spreading rapidly and entering numerous other species suggests that bird flu may soon evolve to produce a human pandemic. According to a recent survey, 56% of U.S. doctors now believe that a global influenza pandemic will arrive sometime in the next four years. The emergence of a possibly catastrophic human influenza pandemic is imminent.

The spread of H5N1 bird flu presents an enormous challenge to futurists charged with anticipating the possible impacts posed by this threat. The stakes are high. According to the United Nations, a bird flu pandemic could kill between 5 million and 150 million people worldwide. The large discrepancy between those two figures reflects the tremendous difference that preparation could play in facing a global pandemic. Fatality rates will vary depending on the strength of the resources that the national health institutions have in place.

Although the developed world is marshaling considerable resources to combat H5N1 bird flu, future flu pandemics will place human health at risk across the globe. Accurate predictions regarding the scope and characteristics of a potential bird flu pandemic may avert a crisis and promote the type of farsighted efforts required to develop and implement improved protection of the public health.

A Brief Overview of Bird Flu

Influenza is a viral respiratory disease that occurs in humans and animals such as pigs, ducks, and chickens. In humans, the symptoms of influenza include fever (possibly severe), muscle aches, and breathing difficulty. Flu is a seasonal disease in the temperate latitudes, with annual infections peaking predictably during the winter months.

The H5N1 bird flu contains two critical viral proteins common to influenza virus strains: hemagglutinin (H) and neuraminidase (N). During infection, the hemagglutinin protein serves as the virus's fuse. It is responsible for the initial infection and entry of the virus

Originally published in the Setpember-October 2006 issue of *The Futurist*. Used with permission from the World Future Society, 7910 Woodmont Avenue, Suite 450, Bethesda, Maryland 20814. Telephone: 301/656-8274; Fax: 301/951-0394; http://www.wfs.org.

into the host cell. The neuraminidase protein acts like gunpowder in a stick of dynamite; it kicks in at the end of the reproduction cycle to spread the newly formed viruses to other cells. By monitoring the exact subtype of H and N proteins found in viruses causing human influenza, health organizations can determine when new forms of the flu virus are emerging.

The avian influenza (H5N1) that has emerged recently is spreading across the world, possibly by wild aquatic birds such as ducks and geese. Bird flu has not infected many humans as yet, but for those few recognized cases the fatality rate has been extremely high. For example, in Vietnam, the fatality rate for reported cases of H5N1 bird flu was 47.5%; Indonesia, 55.6%; and Thailand, 65%, according to the University of Minnesota's Center for Infectious Disease Research and Policy.

> Bird flu has not infected many humans as yet, but for those few recognized cases the fatality rate has been extremely high.

Bird flu seems to involve humans by direct contact, and the concern is that the process of mutation will create a form of bird flu (or something novel) that will readily infect humans by the respiratory route. That might mark the start of a deadly pandemic.

What makes the H5N1 bird flu strain so dangerous is that, not only does it attack the immune system and respiratory system, but it does so with far greater intensity and lethality than common flu. It can move quicker through the body and is less easily stopped.

Precisely how the virus kills remains a mystery to experts and historians. To date, there have been few bird flu infections of humans—217 cases since 2003, according to the World Health Organization (WHO)—but 123 of these cases resulted in death.

The Impacts of Bird Flu on the Poultry Industry

A bird flu pandemic would have tremendous financial costs. That H5N1 has already resulted in the destruction of hundreds of millions of animals, with attendant massive economic losses, is widely known. Poultry production makes up anywhere from 0.6% to 2% of the GDP in East Asian countries. After the 2003 bird flu outbreak in Vietnam, poultry production was down by 15% or about $50 million for that year. If similar declines hit Indonesia, the costs could reach as high as $500 million just in the field of poultry farming.

Many of the world's chicken and poultry farmers are taking steps to prevent their flocks from being infected with bird flu, but it remains to be seen whether—and for how long—such measures can stave off poultry epidemics. Keeping commercial flocks away from wild birds, particularly migratory waterfowl such as ducks (which act as both influenza virus reservoirs and disseminators) is critical.

In addition to keeping domestic and wild birds physically separated, producers of poultry-related goods must also ensure that water and food sources remain uncontaminated. Aquatic waterfowl shed large amounts of virus in their feces and will rapidly introduce influenza into water sources. If domestic birds consume water from the same source contacted by wild waterfowl, chances for the flu to spread to the flock are high. The need to keep flocks separated completely from wild birds may significantly curtail the availability of "free range" animals.

Because H5N1 bird flu is now considered ineradicable in wild populations, it will pose a permanent risk to commercial flocks.

In the aftermath of a deadly bird flu pandemic, the public may become apprehensive about consuming poultry products. We have been unknowingly eating poultry harboring avian influenza viruses for years, but these viruses were not dangerous to humans. The arrival of the deadly H5N1 bird flu is going to change things. The fact that it has been transmitted and caused severe, often lethal, infections in people who have handled diseased animals will cause understandable apprehension and probably some level of consumer avoidance of poultry. Although producers will cull and destroy infected animals, minimizing the chances for any exposure to the consuming public, perceptions and fears may be difficult to control.

Large-scale animal husbandry practices ("factory farming") may increase the likelihood of pandemic. The mass-production methods used by the international poultry industry, such as keeping large numbers of animals in close proximity, could increase the opportunity for transmission. Meat packing, poultry packing, and poultry storage facilities should be carefully watched and managed in order to minimize future global health issues.

Rapid Response Required

One of the most crucial first steps in protecting the public from the threat of a bird flu pandemic is ensuring that health organizations respond quickly and effectively to tips and information they receive about possible small outbreaks of the disease. This information could come in the form of farmers or ranchers reporting illnesses among their flocks to health officials, perhaps through veterinarians. Health officials must act quickly to determine if the illness is a flu and if it is of the deadly H5N1 variety. This is what WHO refers to as "influenza surveillance."

Unfortunately, influenza surveillance is an especially weak link in the chain of public-health protection. Exactly where, when, and (most important) how quickly and reliably the emergence of a new flu virus with pandemic potential is recognized will determine whether a vaccine can be produced before the virus spreads across the world. People and products now traverse the planet with ease, meaning that a future flu pandemic may engulf the world with unprecedented speed.

WHO conducts continuous worldwide surveillance to monitor influenza and detect newly emerging virus subtypes. Despite impressive efforts, the fact that the entire globe must be monitored continuously suggests that coverage in some regions is less than perfect. In the near term, the best chance to control a pandemic is to recognize its emergence as early as possible. This will demand resources sufficient to enable comprehensive, continuous worldwide surveillance and accurate clinical assessments.

Quick culling (slaughter) of infected animals and development of new animal vaccination methods for bird flocks are not necessarily simple or complete solutions. Vaccinations prevent disease, not infection. Although inhibited, H5N1 bird flu viruses might reproduce without generating any obvious signs in vaccinated flocks. Bird vaccinations might interfere with the ability of health workers to determine whether or not the virus is spreading, because both vaccinated birds and sick birds could test positive for flu antibodies. It may be possible to produce a bird flu vaccine that allows health researchers to distinguish between these two groups.

Challenges for Vaccine Production and Distribution

Beyond surveillance, the issue of vaccination—developing a vaccine and making it readily available to several million people—is one of great importance. Proper vaccination of national populations is the most reliable and effective way to limit a bird flu pandemic's destructive scope.

One fear among health officials is that a killer flu might emerge and spread far faster than humanity can manufacture vaccine stocks.

One fear among health officials is that a killer flu might emerge and spread far faster than humanity can manufacture vaccine stocks. Also, there is no certainty that a new pandemic virus would follow the same pattern of previous viruses—a strong upsurge during the winter months, dying off significantly during the spring. History has shown that a pandemic could start well outside of the regular flu season. The great killer flu of 1918 began months earlier than normal.

Unfortunately, these fears are quite credible. If the H5N1 bird flu sparks a human pandemic in the near term, world vaccine supplies will not be able to meet the demand even in a best-case scenario. In a worst-case scenario, no vaccine will be available at all; the world will be in serious trouble.

Vaccine production is more complicated than simple drug production: Producers would need nine months to develop and test virus seed stocks, confirm safety and effectiveness in patient target groups, and scale up vaccine production to meet the needs of entire national populations. The only way to ensure that the vaccine will work against the pandemic strain is to produce it immediately after the new virus has emerged. This means significant casualties may occur before the pandemic is recognized and the large-scale vaccine production process can even begin.

The problem, however, does not end if and when a vaccine stock sufficient to protect everyone from H5N1 bird flu infection is in hand. Hopefully, the ability of national and international health organizations to devise, test, license, and distribute vaccines will improve before a crisis, but a sustained and multifaceted effort will be needed to control the future threat of pandemic influenza.

Both vaccine-development methods and vaccination techniques must be updated and improved to meet a threat that will never recede. One problem with influenza vaccination as practiced now is that the immunity doesn't last long—about two years at most. That means that all of us who stood in line in 1976 to get the free swine flu vaccine are no longer guaranteed protection against that virus if it reemerges. Recent research has indicated that under-the-skin injections, rather than inoculation in muscle tissue, may lead to far more effective vaccination while using less medicine.

Existing influenza vaccine production methods are slow, and we cannot rely on them indefinitely. Pandemics may emerge at any time and anywhere and are projected to spread rapidly. Consequently, depending on vaccines that will be produced using methods that will require months to gear up to the challenge is a risky proposition.

Existing influenza vaccine production methods are slow, and we cannot rely on them indefinitely.

Special Aspects of a Global Disease

Influenza is a winter season disease in temperate latitudes, but it is present year-round in tropical areas. If a pandemic emerged in southern China during the late summer months, vaccine production for the upcoming winter season would already be well under way. The sudden appearance of a new and different virus would require an abrupt shift in vaccine production priorities. Unless this new virus threat were recognized immediately and manufacturing processes were flexible enough to shift quickly to production of the pandemic vaccine, there would be no vaccine ready to meet demand.

The constant challenge posed by flu viruses—their adaptability, hardiness, and capacity for change and explosive emergence—suggests that health organizations should focus on new and faster vaccine production methods. Several technologies, such as cell-culture-based and DNA vaccines, have shown potential and offer promising leads for future development.

Whatever method is used to create the vaccine, planners should keep in mind that pharmaceutical companies are increasingly unwilling to produce these vital drugs without governmental protection from liability litigation. During the 1976 swine flu outbreak, there were a number of deaths from reactions to the vaccine. Since then, vaccine producers have insisted that the potential burden of liability from vaccine-related complications be shared. This could be a significant financial commitment if vaccine is needed for the majority of the population. News coverage of President Bush's $7.1 billion budget for avian flu protection frequently fails to mention the potential cost of litigation protection.

WHO's GUIDELINES FOR RECOGNIZING PANDEMIC

In April 2006, the World Health Organization reissued these guidelines to humanitarian agencies for recognizing and planning for outbreaks.

INTER-PANDEMIC PERIOD

Phase 1. No new influenza virus subtypes have been detected in humans, but a new strain of the virus may have caused infection in animals. The risk to humans is considered to be low.

Public-Health Goal: Strengthen influenza pandemic preparedness at the global, regional, national, and subnational levels.

Phase 2. A circulating animal influenza virus subtype poses a substantial risk of human disease. However, no new influenza virus subtypes have been detected in humans.

Public-Health Goal: Minimize the risk of transmission to humans, and work to detect and report any transmissions quickly after they occur.

PANDEMIC ALERT PERIOD

Phase 3. A human infection with a new influenza virus subtype has been documented, but little or no human-to-human spread has occurred.

Public-Health Goal: Categorize the new virus subtype to aid early detection efforts. Quickly respond to and publicize any new cases.

Phase 4. Small clusters of outbreaks have developed with limited human-to-human transmission. The spread is highly localized. This suggests that the new influenza strain is not well adapted to humans.

Public Health Goal: Contain the new virus within a limited area, work to delay spread of virus, and implement preparedness measures, including vaccine development.

Phase 5. Larger clusters of influenza-stricken patients have appeared, but the spread is still localized, suggesting that the virus is adapting to humans but may not be fully transmissible. A substantial risk for pandemic is associated with this phase.

Public Health Goal: Maximize efforts to contain the virus to a specific location, with the understanding that a pandemic could be imminent.

PANDEMIC PERIOD

Phase 6. Increased and sustained transmission of deadly virus to the general population.

Public-Health Goal: Minimize the impact of the pandemic through such measures as social distancing and use of face masks.

Source: Pandemic Influenza Preparedness and Mitigation in Refugee and Displaced Populations WHO Guidelines for Humanitarian Agencies. The World Health Organization, 2006. Further information is available at NTD Information Resource Centre, World Health Organization, 1211 Geneva 27, Switzerland. E-mail ntddocs@who.int.

Although stockpiling anti-influenza drugs like Tamiflu is an important strategy to augment vaccination during high-demand episodes or hedge against the possibility that no vaccines will be available to meet demands, this is not a final solution to the pandemic influenza problem. If a pandemic strikes in the near term, the capacity to manufacture vaccine will not be sufficient to meet the enormous upsurge in worldwide demand. Influenza viruses exhibit a prodigious capacity to adapt, and it seems likely that extensive use of any compound like Tamiflu will quickly result in the creation of mutant, Tamiflu-resistant influenza viruses. For example, the influenza viruses that were common last season are now resistant to anti-influenza agents used against them.

Tamiflu stockpiling, producing vaccine seed stocks before a crisis, and obtaining more ventilators to support large numbers of patients during outbreaks are all simultaneously crucial and comforting steps, but they do not ensure complete and permanent protection from pandemic. A full-scale outbreak will quickly overwhelm medical facilities and staff, deplete drug stockpiles, and disrupt civic functions.

Despite the rapid spread and potential deadliness of H5N1 bird flu, there is no certainty that this particular strain of influenza will actually cause a great human pandemic. What is certain, however, is that several separate subforms of H5N1 influenza have appeared and are evolving in birds. At the same time, other new types of bird flu viruses with entirely different H and N proteins have also emerged. Even in the unlikely event that H5N1 bird flu disappeared suddenly, we would still not be safe, because the basic biology of influenza is unchangeable; thus, the underlying conditions that could lead to a pandemic would remain in place.

Past experience suggests that the sequence of events culminating in a pandemic is rare. As both human and food animal populations expand, and methods are altered to meet burgeoning worldwide demand for cattle and poultry products, we must be alert to the fact that large-scale poultry-packing facilities may be ground zero for virus evolution and transmission. Researchers have also considered that humans will have more of a hand in starting a future pandemic than is generally appreciated.

In short, pandemic influenza should be viewed as a permanent problem that can only be managed, but never solved definitively.

ABSENTEEISM IN THE WAKE OF OUTBREAK

In the event of an influenza pandemic, public-health employees are the public's first and most important line of defense. But more than 40% of health-care employees say they would stay home if a flu pandemic hit.

Doctors and nurses were the least likely to skip work during a pandemic, but technical and support staff—necessary for launching a coordinated bird-flu response—were two to three times less likely to report for duty. Only 26% of technical or support staff believed it was likely they would even be called to work by their health departments in the event of a pandemic, a recent survey by the Johns Hopkins Bloomberg School of Public Health revealed.

According to the survey, administrative personnel who understood how vital they were to the response effort were far more likely to indicate that they would show up for work during a global flu crisis. Frighteningly, only 15.1% of the technical and support staff the researchers interviewed felt that they had an important role in the agency.

To address this problem, the researchers recommend that health-care managers communicate to their technical and administrative workers that they are indeed essential to the public's response to any outbreak.

The costs of medical care could, according to some, reach $100 to $200 billion dollars in the United States alone. The Web site www.Avianinfluenza.org has taken those health figures, applied them to other high-income nations, and determined that the ultimate cost of a pandemic could conceivably reach $550 billion.

Outside of hospitals, a pandemic would have an immediate and catastrophic effect on the day-today operations of the world's corporations. But business leaders can lessen the financial disruption by preparing their companies for pandemic, says workplace authority John Challenger.

"Employers will be on the frontline of any outbreak, since business travel and workplaces are major factors in the spread of any virus," says Challenger. "This puts them in a position to either accelerate an outbreak or help prevent one from reaching pandemic proportions. Just a few confirmed or suspected cases of human-to-human transmission of a new flu virus in a city could lead to widespread absenteeism, as parents stay home and take their children out of school in an effort to avoid possible contact with infected people." He estimates that a pandemic could cost the U.S. economy as much as $670 billion.

Workers could unknowingly carry the illness for days and infect those around them. To protect workers—and the bottom line—from the effects of a pandemic, Challenger suggests that employers and managers consider the following:

- Increase the number of shifts. This will reduce the number of people working in the office at any one time.

- Expand personal space. Urge workers to suspend close contact and remain three feet apart from one another at all times.

- Limit meetings. If there is no need to gather large groups of workers in a confined space, then don't do it. Conduct meetings via conference calls. Bigger companies may want to consider video conferencing.

- Have a supply of surgical masks for workers to wear.

- Allow employees to shop online during the day for limited periods, thus helping them to avoid crowded shopping areas.

- Check heating and air-conditioning systems and consider turning these systems off. Heating systems are prime carriers for airborne illnesses like influenza. If it's not possible to turn off the heat or air, make sure that the filters on these systems are cleaned often.

"The best solution may be switching to a predominantly telecommuting workforce. Any employee who can do his or her work from home with a computer and a phone should be doing so prior to an outbreak. This will help prevent a flu virus from spreading among co-workers," Challenger concludes.

Sources: Challenger, Gray & Christmas, 150 South Wacker Drive, 27th Floor, Chicago, Illinois 60606. Telephone 312-332-5790; Web site www.challengergray.com.

The Johns Hopkins University Public Affairs Office, 615 North Wolfe Street, W1600, Baltimore, Maryland 21205. Telephone 410-955-6878; Web site wwwjhu.edu.

Panic Attack

By William Speed Weed
Current Science, January 20, 2006

It's almost impossible to open a newspaper or turn on the TV news nowadays without encountering a headline about avian influenza. Better known as bird flu, the disease has killed tens of millions of chickens in Asia. So far, only about 120 people have caught bird flu, but half of them have died.

A climate of fear over bird flu has spread faster than the disease itself. Many journalists and medical authorities have sounded an alarm that the disease could soon become a human pandemic—a worldwide epidemic. One scientist called avian flu "the single greatest risk to our world today."

Other authorities say such claims are overblown. "You just can't say this thing's going to tear off and take us all down," says one skeptic, Earl Brown, a professor of microbiology at the University of Ottawa. "There's a lot of biology in between."

The "Biology in Between"

Bird flu is caused by a virus, H5N1, first discovered in Scotland in 1959. Viruses are tiny life-forms that reside in one type of animal and normally do little harm. H5N1 is native to the intestines of ducks. It doesn't kill ducks because it needs them to survive. If it killed a lot of ducks, it would have no place to live.

Occasionally, a virus jumps to a new species that has no immunity, or natural defense, against it. Human immunodeficiency virus (HIV), the virus that causes acquired immune deficiency syndrome (AIDS), jumped from chimpanzees to humans in the late 1970s. HIV is deadly to humans who don't receive treatment, because we have developed no immunity to it.

H5N1 has leapt from ducks to chickens and is killing them in large numbers. H5N1 could also infect many humans, Brown concedes, but would first have to undergo two changes.

When H5N1 invades the human body, it resides deep in the lungs, where it provokes a furious immune reaction that can be fatal. But the virus's residence in the lower lungs also makes it less transmissible—capable of being passed to other organisms. A sneeze won't expel H5N1 particles into the air. So H5N1 is extremely lethal but cannot move from person to person through the air.

Those two traits are two strikes against bird flu's becoming a serious threat, says Brown. A virus that can't be transmitted easily from person to person can't lead to a pandemic. Neither can one that is so deadly. But aren't pandemics supposed to be deadly? Yes, but a virus's goal is not to kill its host but to survive and reproduce. H5N1's current human mortality rate is 50 percent—it kills one out of every two people it infects. A virus that kills so many hosts can't thrive and expand its range.

Ten years ago, Ebola hemorrhagic fever created a media scare. Ebola is a gruesome viral disease that originated in Africa. The best-selling book The Hot Zone, by Richard Preston, asserted that the United States had barely avoided an Ebola epidemic. But Ebola's mortality rate is almost 100 percent. Its extremely deadly nature limits its ability to spread through the human population.

Change in Behavior

To become pandemic, says Brown, H5N1 must evolve two new and separate traits—higher transmissibility and lower mortality. Viruses certainly do evolve; they mutate, or undergo a change in their genetic makeup. A mutation can lead to a change in the virus's behavior. A mutated H5N1 that is capable of residing in the upper lungs instead of the lower lungs would be more transmissible. But mutations are random, says Brown. A virus doesn't choose how it changes. It mutates only as a result of haphazard mistakes in its chemistry.

So H5N1 could mutate, becoming both more transmissible and less deadly. But the likelihood of that happening is comparable to winning the lottery twice, says Brown.

Wanted: Investigators

That said, a global pandemic of some kind is, in all likelihood, on its way. Millions of influenza viruses exist in the world. Perhaps right now, a virus that is completely off scientists' radar screens is developing mutations that will allow it to leap into humans and kill millions of us. Pandemics break out about three times per century. The Spanish flu pandemic of 1918–1919 killed 25 million to 50 million people.

No one should panic about H5N1, but medical authorities should be constantly on the lookout for the next pandemic, says Shelley Hearne of the Trust for America's Health. Brown agrees. If we start to see a cluster of lethal viral infections spreading directly from person to person in, say, Africa or Asia, then we should start to worry.

Is the United States prepared for a pandemic? No, says Hearne. A recently announced plan by the Bush administration to stockpile antiviral drugs and establish a pandemic preparedness program is a good first step, she says. "But what we really need is people," she told *Current Science*. "Another major pandemic will hit us, probably in the lifetime of your readers. And we just don't have the virologists and the epidemiologists [people who study how diseases move through populations] to stay one step ahead.

"Think of Mother Nature as the murderer she sometimes is. What we need more than anything is the scientists who are going to be the CSI detectives figuring out what the next pandemic will be and how to fight it when it comes."

HOW FLU DRUGS WORK

1. When a flu virus invades a cell in the body, the virus multiplies. Now viruses bud from the surface of the cell, and proteins cut the budding viruses free, allowing them to invade and infect other cells.

2. Flu drugs reduce the severity of human flu strains if taken within two days of the appearance of the first symptoms. Bird flu patients may need earlier and larger doses.

3. The drugs disable the proteins that cut the budding viruses from infected cells. Unable to escape, the viruses can't invade new cells, and the infection is stalled.

What the President Should Have Said About Bird Flu

By Nick Schulz
The Saturday Evening Post, January/February 2006

Stung by criticism over the unpreparedness of government at all levels to address Hurricane Katrina, President Bush has been taking steps to make sure another disaster doesn't embarrass his administration. When Hurricane Rita formed in the Gulf, the White House was noticeably more active prior to that storm's landfall. Recently, President Bush addressed in extensive detail at a press conference his thoughts about the threat of an avian flu pandemic.

"If we had an outbreak somewhere in the United States," Bush said, "do we not then quarantine that part of the country, and how do you then enforce a quarantine? . . . And who best to be able to affect a quarantine? One option is the use of a military that's able to plan and move."

So the President has given some thought to what could be a serious problem—the virus, H5N1, has already killed up to 100 people in Asia. Estimates vary, but a global outbreak could kill as many as 150 million people. Papers published recently in the journals *Nature* and *Science* from researchers at the Armed Forces Institute of Pathology, the Centers for Disease Control and Prevention, and Mount Sinai School of Medicine suggest the flu could be more catastrophic than previously thought.

While quarantines need to be considered, they are difficult to execute effectively in countries like the United States that are large and have a diverse and highly mobile population.

A better idea is to take steps to make sure a quarantine isn't necessary. One idea that health and government experts now seem to agree on is the need to stockpile the antiviral treatment Tamiflu. Jeffrey Levi of Trust for America's Health, a nongovernmental organization (NGO), told the AP, "It appears that this is the only effective intervention we have once someone has been infected." Doctors in Asia are already using it to combat bird flu.

There's one big problem, however—there's not a lot of Tamiflu to go around these days. It takes a long time to manufacture the drug, and as governments and health agencies seek to procure it, they're finding they have to wait.

President Bush hinted at this problem in his press conference. "One of the issues is how do we encourage the manufacturing capacity of the country," Bush said, " . . . to be prepared to deal with the outbreak of a pandemic? In other words, can we surge enough production to be able to help deal with the issue?"

Presently the answer is no.

The drug was invented by Gilead Sciences of California, and they licensed manufacturing and distribution rights to Roche, the Swiss drug giant. But even though Tamiflu has been known as an effective treatment against H5N1 for several years, Roche presently lacks the capacity to fill orders quickly.

According to a report in *Business Week*, the Secretary of the Department of Health and Human Services, Mike Leavitt, wants a stockpile capable of treating 20 million Americans. Currently the U.S. can treat just over 2 million people. But an order placed by

---

"Right now, our national stockpiles of antiviral drugs sit at dangerously low levels—about 2 percent of what we would need in a serious outbreak."—Senator Bill Frist

---

American officials for another 3 million treatments will only be filled by Roche in 2006. Senator Bill Frist, who has taken a keen interest in the issue, recently called the supply for Americans "totally inadequate."

"Right now, our national stockpiles of antiviral drugs sit at dangerously low levels—about 2 percent of what we would need in a serious outbreak," Frist wrote recently in the *Washington Times*.

And it's not just the United States that's waiting. "It will take Roche two years to complete the United Kingdom's stockpile order to treat 14.6 million of its citizens," *Business Week* reports. The writer and blogger Randall Parker has created an invaluable overview of the stockpiling efforts of several nations. He illustrates the gravity of the situation by pointing out that the World Health Organization—the global body responsible for coordinating the counterattack on a flu pandemic—won't even have a few million doses until the middle of 2006. Today it only has 80,000.

Supply is so tight, *ABC News* reports, that Roche has had to institute a "first-come, first-serve" waiting list. Unfortunately for Americans, "the United States is nowhere near the top of that list."

The capacity situation is bad enough that Gilead sued to force Roche to relinquish manufacturing rights to the drug in the hopes that it will be able to massively ramp up production.

So here's one area where President Bush could take some proactive steps. According to the *San Francisco Chronicle*, Roche is planning to build a plant in the United States, but it would not be producing drugs until the end of 2006. To speed things up, President Bush could order the Food and Drug Administration to speed up approval of other, already established plants in the United States for manufacturing the ingredients of Tamillu. The FDA has taken similar steps in response to infectious disease outbreaks, such as its efforts to fast-track available treatments for HIV/AIDS.

And President Bush could encourage Roche to initiate a technology transfer to manufacturers in the U.S. to ramp up development. This would respect the property and contract rights enjoyed by Roche while getting more product to the clinics, hospitals and programs that need it.

George Mason University economist Tyler Cowen, who established an avian flu website to track the disease, also suggests stockpiling "high-quality masks and antibiotics for secondary infections (often more dangerous than the flu itself) and, more important, have a good plan for distribution and dealing with extraordinary excess demand and possibly panic."

Lastly, Tamiflu is an important part in a first-line defense against a flu pandemic—Sen. Frist pointed out that if an outbreak occurs, "Tamiflu is what people would go after. It's what you're going to ask for, I'm going to ask for, immediately." But it is no cure-all. Work needs to proceed on vaccines, as well as procurement of other possible treatments, like an injectable form of the drug Relenza, made by GlaxoSmithKline, especially as there may be instances of resistance to Tamiflu if it is used widely.

President Bush shouldn't be focusing on a quarantine just yet. He should be taking steps to make sure a quarantine isn't necessary. He has outlined some steps to do that. But if he has learned anything from Katrina, he can demonstrate it by taking steps to make sure that, while the United States is presently "nowhere near the top of the list" for the treatments needed to fight an outbreak, that situation doesn't last long.

Spreading Its Wings

By Nancy Shute
U.S. News & World Report, March 20, 2006

Steven Hinrichs delights in watching the sandhill cranes that soar along Nebraska's Platte River each March on their spring migration north. This year, that delight has turned to dread. Hinrichs directs the University of Nebraska's Center for Biosecurity, and he knows that birds can bring not only beauty but also death. "I don't think it's a coincidence," he says, that the 1918 flu pandemic, which killed perhaps 50 million people worldwide, originated nearby.

Nebraska is on the famed Central Flyway, a route that millions of birds follow each year as they migrate from southern wintering grounds north to Alaska and the Arctic to breed. While there, the birds often mingle with birds from Asia, where H5N1 avian flu, widely regarded as the bug most likely to mutate and spark a human pandemic, is rampant. When the sandhills return in the fall, Hinrichs wonders, "what will they bring back?"

He's not the only one asking that question. David Nabarro, the United Nations' bird flu czar, said last week that he expects bird flu to reach the Americas in a migratory bird in the next six to 12 months. Federal agencies announced ramped-up efforts to detect H5N1 in wild birds. "We expect H5N1 to arrive in the United States," Agriculture Secretary Michael Johanns told *U.S. News* last week. "If migratory birds can spread it, and we're heading into spring, we need to be prepared." The goal is to create a system to detect the virus's entry into North America early on. With more notice, infectious disease specialists hope they can slow the contagion among wild birds and poultry, thus reducing odds that it will jump to humans or, in the worst case, mutate and gain the ability to spread from human to human, setting off a deadly pandemic. Even without a pandemic, the advent of H5N1 could have enormous economic impact. Although only one commercial poultry farm in Europe has been infected, poultry sales there have plummeted as much as 70 percent in the past month—even though eating cooked chicken doesn't pose any risk.

Starting in April, researchers from several federal agencies will test roughly 100,000 birds, dead and alive, as well as bird feces, in Alaska, Hawaii, and the lower 48. The survey was launched in 1996; this year's endeavor will test eight times as many birds as in the previous years combined. The samples will be run through a network of 39 federal, state, and university laboratories equipped to do rapid polymerase-chain-reaction testing, which copies bits of DNA, and can handle 18,000 samples a day, part of a national laboratory upgrade funded by post-9/11 federal bioterrorism programs.

Natural Step. "There's little question in my mind that we will at some point see a wild bird [with H5N1] enter our domain," says Michael Leavitt, secretary of health and human services, who convened summits last week with officials in North Dakota and South Dakota to discuss pandemic flu preparations. "We don't view that as a crisis; we see that as a natural step along the path. It would not be unusual, seeing what's happening in the rest of the world." As part of its pandemic flu precautions, the United States is buying 19.5 million courses of antiviral drugs, but no one knows if they will work against H5N1. The feds are also testing experimental vaccines, but because domestic vaccine production facilities are lacking, it will take at least six months from the start of a pandemic to make significant amounts. Thus, the hope that surveillance will bring early warning and more time to mount a response.

> At least 97 people are known to have died from bird flu since 2003. Almost all of them lived in households with backyard poultry flocks.

The need for surveillance, a time-honored technique in infectious disease control, is particularly acute because no one knows exactly how the H5N1 virus has spread so far, so fast. Avian influenza has been around for at least a century in both wild and domesticated birds. But until recently, outbreaks of virulent strains in poultry were exceedingly rare. The H5N1 virus first appeared in 1997, when thousands of chickens in Hong Kong suddenly sickened and died. That outbreak was halted when public-health officials ordered the slaughter of all the poultry in Hong Kong. The virus re-emerged in Southeast Asia in 2003 and proliferated rapidly. That outbreak continues, and efforts to contain it by culling flocks or vaccinating birds, measures that had worked in the past, have failed. At least 97 people are known to have died from bird flu since 2003. Almost all of them lived in households with backyard poultry flocks.

But in the past year, avian influenza has started to kill wild birds, which had long been able to harbor the disease without getting sick. In April 2005, more than 6,000 bar-headed geese died at Qinghai Lake in central China, a congregating point for migratory fowl. That was a wake-up call to wildlife biologists; the last time avian influenza afflicted large numbers of wildfowl was in 1961. "That's the really surprising part of it, that wild birds are now being killed by this virus as well," says Leslie Dierauf, director of the USGS National Wildlife Health Center in Madison, Wis. "It's changed somehow, and we're not sure how."

Indeed, three months after the Qinghai Lake die-off, poultry in Western Siberia started dying of H5N1. The virus has spread like wildfire since then, first moving through Central Asia into Turkey and eastern Europe. Those viruses, when tested, proved almost identical to those recovered from the birds at Qinghai Lake.

In the past three months, the H5N1 virus has gone ballistic, infecting birds in 21 countries in Africa, Europe, and the Middle East. It's unclear if the outbreaks are the result of bird migrations, poultry shipments, or other human activities. In some countries, like Nigeria, only poultry has been infected. In others, like Germany, only wild birds are dying. The uncertainty has set off a fierce battle between some wildlife conservationists, who feel that wild birds are being unfairly maligned, and agricultural interests.

"Who is the spreader?" asks Robert Webster, a bird flu authority at St. Jude's Children's Research Hospital in Memphis. Webster, working with colleagues in Asia, reported last month that H5N1 is widespread in migratory birds in southern China, suggesting that they could carry the virus long distances. Webster says he's less concerned about the dead birds found in recent weeks in Europe than he is about those still aloft. "Dead birds don't migrate."

Testing Flocks. Commercial poultry growers in the United States are acutely aware of the risk posed by H5N1, not the least because they've been dealing with less lethal and more common forms of bird flu for decades. The highly pathogenic H5 and H7 strains are both rare and more lethal, killing 80 to 100 percent of the birds infected. The United States has had three outbreaks of these strains, in 1924, 1983, and 2004; slaughtering the birds and disinfecting the farms contained them. In 2003, the Netherlands killed more than 30 million birds to arrest an outbreak of H7N7 bird flu. Other countries, notably China, have used vaccines, but the United States and most European nations eschew that method, arguing that vaccinated birds can act as carriers and infect others. If H5N1 attacked U.S. poultry flocks, producers would use the slaughter, quarantine, and sanitation techniques that have worked in the past, says Richard Lobb, a spokesman for the National Chicken Council. Almost all commercial poultry is raised indoors, and in January the large producers, which account for 95 percent of the chicken sold in the United States, started testing all flocks for H5N1.

"The poultry industry in the United States is well prepared to detect and manage an outbreak," says Nina Marano, associate director for veterinary public health for the Centers for Disease Control and Prevention, who specializes in zoonoses, or diseases like

> In the past three months, the H5N1 virus has gone ballistic, infecting birds in 21 countries in Africa, Europe, and the Middle East.

H5N1 and West Nile virus that pass from animals to humans. She frets more about protecting the country's approximately 50,000 hobby flocks, as well as exhibition birds and live poultry markets.

The country's major zoos, which are shelters of last resort for endangered species, and also commonly host chickens, wild ducks, and geese, are buttoning up plans to deal with H5N1. Those range from shutting down walk-through aviaries to quizzing visitors on their recent travels. "You can't eliminate wild birds," says Robyn Barbiers, a veterinarian at Chicago's Lincoln Park Zoo who chairs the American Zoo and Aquarium Association's animal health committee. When West Nile virus arrived in the United States in 1999 and started killing wild birds, everyone was nervous, she says. "We dealt with it," says Barbiers. "I don't think avian influenza is going to be as disastrous as people envision."

But H5N1 could prove disastrous in countries like Nigeria, where the virus has been detected on more than 130 poultry farms in the past month. Webster says when he lies awake worrying, it's about places like Africa where lab capacity, cash, and expertise are all scarce. "I worry that the virus will end up in humans and not necessarily be detected," he says. It would take just one sick person on an overseas flight to ignite a pandemic.

Last week, health officials from around the world met in Geneva to talk about how to stop a pandemic—something that has never been attempted, let alone realized. Intensive surveillance of animal and human flu cases would be essential to containment, providing enough time to vaccinate people and treat them with antivirals before the disease could spread.

Until H5N1, notes Webster, the world wasn't interested in bird flu. "Who gives a damn about a virus that's out there in wild birds and doesn't do anything? Now we know," he says, "that we do have to understand the natural history of these things, because they do have consequences."

Immediate Treatment Needed for Bird Flu Cases, Study Says

By Donald G. McNeil Jr.
The New York Times, September 11, 2006

Avian flu kills in much the same way the global flu pandemic of 1918 did, by drowning victims in fluid produced in their own lungs, a new study has found. The study also suggests that immediate treatment with antiviral drugs is crucial, because the virus reproduces so quickly that, if not suppressed within the first 48 hours, it tends to push victims into a rapid decline to death.

"The paradigm 'hit hard and hit early' probably is very true for H5N1 influenza," said Dr. Menno D. de Jong, an Oxford University virologist and the study's lead author. However, he added, because the body's own immune response does part of the damage, doctors should consider giving anti-inflammatory drugs along with antivirals like Tamiflu.

Although the results of the relatively small study are precisely what flu experts had predicted from laboratory work, Dr. Anne Moscona, a professor of pediatrics and immunology at the Weill Cornell Medical College, called it a "major advance," because so little clinical information had previously been gleaned from the 241 known cases of the disease.

Many of those cases have been in rural villages in Asia, where victims pick it up from backyard chickens and are buried before the virus that killed them is even identified. Provincial hospitals have done few autopsies and little genetic analysis.

This study, which appears in the October issue of Nature Medicine, was led by an Oxford research team in Ho Chi Minh City, Vietnam, and compared 18 people with the A(H5N1) avian flu in 2004 and 2005 to 8 people infected with seasonal human flus.

It found that the avian flu patients, and particularly the 13 who died from it, had unusually high levels of the virus in their bodies. Consequently, they also had high levels of the chemicals, known as cytokines and chemokines, that set off the immune system's inflammatory response.

Those chemicals, some of which are produced in cells lining the narrowest passages in the lungs, draw in white blood cells to attack invaders. But doing so too vigorously can flood the lungs, causing deadly pneumonia.

The effect, known as the "cytokine storm" is the leading theory as to why so many young, previously healthy people died in the 1918–19 pandemic, known as the Spanish flu, which killed tens of millions of people. Seasonal flus tend to kill the very old and very young, who usually die from bacterial infections that develop days after the milder flu virus has irritated their lung tissue.

The avian flu virus was easier to detect in throat swabs than in nasal swabs, Dr. de Jong said, which is the opposite of how seasonal flu is detected, and useful for doctors doing flu tests. And the virus was found in rectal swabs, which is important for hospitals to know because it means diarrhea, common among flu patients, can also spread the disease.

Flu experts were surprised that such high concentrations of the virus were found in nose and throat swabs. Earlier studies had suggested that the avian flu is not easily transmitted between humans because, unlike seasonal flu, it attaches primarily to receptors found deep in the lungs.

Dr. de Jong said there could be several explanations: the throat swabs could have picked up virus coughed up from the lungs. Different receptors are spread up and down the breathing tract. And it is possible—though unproved—that some people may simply be born with receptors more amenable to the virus. That theory has been offered by epidemiologists who note that, even in villages where all the chickens are sick, human outbreaks tend to cluster in families.

The study also showed that some of the flu strains isolated in Vietnam had particular genetic changes that virologists have been watching for, fearing that these changes would make them more lethal.

But those changes appeared in only some patients, and in those who died as well as those who lived, "so I wouldn't make too much of it," Dr. Moscona said.

Henry L. Niman, a Pittsburgh biochemist who has been tracking viral changes and raised earlier alarms about E627K, agreed.

"Lethality in the virus may rely on several changes," he said. "But it's got several different paths to the same end. That's what makes it so efficient."

IV. The Psychological and Economic Impact of Epidemics

Editor's Introduction

Should the avian flu or another aggressively virulent disease develop into a pandemic in the near future, world governments and the global medical community have a comprehensive understanding of what would be needed to counteract it. Drugs would have to be produced on a massive scale. Medical workers and care facilities would need to be mobilized. Quarantines might also have to be implemented to isolate the afflicted from the healthy. However, no one can truly anticipate the psychological and economic impact a global epidemic would have on society at large. During the Spanish Flu pandemic of 1918–19, people wore gauze masks and refrained from gathering in large groups. In certain areas businesses either closed or asked customers to place their orders outside their stores. Health-care workers, themselves often suffering from the flu, were spread too thin to adequately care for the afflicted. Moreover, in certain regions there were not enough grave diggers to bury the dead, so the deceased were interred by steam shovel in mass graves, often without coffins. Commerce suffered, as did the psychological well being of the survivors, as many were mentally scarred by the experience of seeing so many young and healthy people succumb to the disease.

Today, when modern jet planes and ships can transport people and products across the world far more efficiently than in the first quarter of the 20th century, when the average person travels farther and more often than his grandparents did, the fear exists that a pandemic could spread far more widely and quickly than at any other point in our history. No one can predict what such an outbreak would do to the global economy, nor can anyone anticipate the sort of emotional damage it would inflict on our collective psyche. The entries in this section set aside the medical repercussions of an epidemic to explore the possible psychological and economic trauma it could cause.

In the first article, "The Fear Factor," Nancy Shute reports on the current efforts of international bodies such as the World Health Organization to inform people about the risks of an epidemic flu outbreak without causing a panic. Writing for *Modern Healthcare*, Cinda Becker discusses the economic impact on health-care providers and suppliers that a flu pandemic could have. Though normal flu outbreaks boost hospital admissions (and profits) seasonally, a pandemic could easily overtax the system.

In "Three Things You Don't Know About AIDS in Africa," Emily Oster, offers an unconventional perspective on the crisis, one that suggests we change the way we think about the disease in order to stifle its further spread. In another look at AIDS, "The HIV Trade-Off," David Batstone describes the economics of the epidemic, noting how some have questioned whether it is cost-effective to provide drugs to impoverished victims in Africa.

The final article in this section, "Death by Mosquito," by Christine Gorman, discusses the global impact of malaria on the economy and asks why more isn't being done to effectively combat this curable disease.

The Fear Factor

By Nancy Shute
U.S. News & World Report, November 21, 2005

A disease outbreak that could happen 30 years from now isn't at the top of most people's list of worries. But now the deadly avian flu virus has leapt from Asia into Europe, and perhaps the Middle East. President Bush is talking about how the military could help quarantine victims of a flu pandemic. And new United Nations pandemic flu czar David Nabarro cautions that up to 150 million people could die. Influenza is, suddenly, a source of great fear.

That's good news to infectious disease experts in the United States and abroad, who since 1997 have warned that the newly emerged H5N1 strain of bird flu posed a serious threat of sparking a human pandemic, only to have those warnings largely ignored. But it's bad news, too. Their worry is that this spike in public concern will soon wane but the threat will not, leaving nations and families unprepared. Thus the dilemma: How do you tell people to prepare for a risk that may be horrendous, but maybe not? For the first time, figuring out what to tell people, and when, has become a major part of preparing for a disaster, be it a Category 5 hurricane, a bioterrorism attack, or a deadly new strain of flu.

Tricky. "We've really been walking a tightrope on pandemic communications," says Dick Thompson, spokesman for infectious disease with the World Health Organization in Geneva. "We've wanted to motivate countries into action, but we haven't wanted to sacrifice our credibility with scare tactics. We don't know the timing of the next pandemic, how severe it will be. We don't know what drugs will work. We don't have a vaccine. Yet we're telling them to prepare for a pandemic. It's tricky." It's even trickier because some WHO members are not known for their candor—China, which tried to suppress news of the 2003 SARS outbreak, comes to mind. But during last week's meeting in Geneva to map a pandemic strategy, WHO membership backed the new, blunt approach. "This is scary, and we don't know," says Thompson. "That's the message."

The U.S. Department of Health and Human Services, which just four years ago was insisting that a Florida man's anthrax infection couldn't possibly be due to terrorism, is also learning the virtues of uncertainty and trepidation. "If a pandemic hits our shores, it will affect almost every sector of our society, not just healthcare but transportation systems, workplaces, schools, public safety, and more," HHS chief Mike Leavitt said last month. "We are inadequately prepared."

Much of this new willingness to play it straight with the public is due to an evolution in the understanding of how people communicate important but upsetting information—and how easily that communication can go awry. In the past 40 years, the analysis of risk has grown into a science, increasingly relied on by businesses and government in deciding how to spend their billions of dollars more wisely or profitably, be it on new cancer treatments or hurricane-resistant buildings. But where risk assessment is mathematical and quantifiable, risk communication is subtle and often counterintuitive.

Panic. For instance, public officials often presume that people will panic when told of impending disaster. So they overdo their efforts to reassure them, which paradoxically prompts people to panic. Dur-

> "The public can generally tolerate much higher levels of alarm than politicians imagine."— Peter Sandman, Rutgers University professor

ing the disastrous 1918 flu pandemic, which killed at least 50 million people worldwide, U.S. officials were obsessed with preserving morale and never publicly acknowledged that the deadly flu outbreaks posed a danger. Near anarchy ensued, with people afraid to go to work or tend to the sick. Dead bodies were left in the streets, and orphans were abandoned. "You will only get panic if people lose faith in their own authorities," says Baruch Fischhoff, a psychologist at Carnegie Mellon University who researches risk communication. "They'll lose faith much quicker if the authorities don't level with them."

That lesson has been hard for nations to learn, even in recent times. In 2003, for example, Chinese officials scrambled to hide reports of a pneumonialike outbreak in Guangdong province. Their secretiveness is widely thought to have given the SARS virus time to spread beyond China, eventually infecting 8,000 people, killing 800, and bringing the Asian economy to a standstill. In October 2001, Tommy Thompson, then secretary of HHS, told an American public still reeling from 9/11 that a Florida man's anthrax infection appeared to be "an isolated case," perhaps contracted by drinking from a stream. Four more people died; the U.S. Capitol was shut down, and people swamped doctors' offices seeking the antibiotic Cipro. Even when no one is harmed, risk-communication failures destroy trust. Tom Ridge, the first secretary of homeland security, will be forever remembered for the department's widely mocked color-coded terror alerts. "The public can generally tolerate much higher levels of alarm than politicians imagine," says Peter Sandman, a Rutgers University professor and risk communications consultant.

Misunderstanding. Risk is a subjective concept. People are usually more worried about risks that are new, unfair, or forced upon them—say, having a toxic-waste dump put next to their home. But people tend to get less upset about risks that are familiar or that they take on of their own volition, like smoking or driving on the interstate. These mundane risks cause far more illness, injury, and death than all toxic-waste sites combined. Armed with data, some risk analysts call those kinds of responses irrational, revealing a yawning gulf of misunderstanding between technocrats and those in harm's way. "The tendency to say the public disagrees because they're ignorant is not fair or correct," says Paul Slovic, a psychologist at the University of Oregon and a pioneer in studying risk perception. "Risk lives in our minds not just as calculations but as

---

Preparing for a pandemic is problematic because
even the experts don't know when it will hit or how
bad it will be.

---

feelings. That's how we navigate through life."

Finding out how people feel about a distressing subject like pandemic flu, Slovic says, is critical if you want them to listen. Scientists, unfortunately, are inclined to think of communication as a science lesson: how avian flu could mutate into a form that would easily infect humans, say, or how nuclear power plants are constructed. The intended audience may be thinking something far different. With Hurricane Katrina, for example, many people refused to evacuate not because they didn't think the hurricane could be deadly but because they didn't want to leave their pets behind.

Obsessed. When people become aware of a threat, they typically seek out information on it and start figuring out what to do. Some might obsess; Internet chat rooms are now awash with people debating the merits of various bird flu treatments or trading tips on how best to heat the house if fuel supplies are interrupted during a pandemic. But in most cases, risk experts say, people soon settle into a "new normal" and get on with life.

Preparing for a pandemic is problematic because even the experts don't know when it will hit or how bad it will be. "The case for taking precautions isn't that you expect the bad outcome," says Sandman, who has advised numerous countries, including the United States, on pandemic communications, "but rather that you can't afford to take the chance, and that it will be too late to protect yourself by the time you know whether the bad outcome is going to happen or not."

Until very recently, the federal government has been loath to scare its citizenry. Its draft pandemic flu plan, unveiled in 2004, talked of only a mild pandemic with 89,000 to 207,000 deaths in the United States, similar to the 1957 and 1968 pandemics. The report included statements that are astonishingly optimistic: "Pandemic influenza can be controlled by rapid, appropriate public-health action that includes surveillance, identification and isolation of influenza cases, infection control, and intense contact tracing. These measures can be a temporary inconvenience to those involved but are essential for containing a pandemic outbreak."

In fact, no pandemic has ever been controlled or contained. Although infectious disease experts are hoping to try to do that using vaccines and antiviral drugs, none of them are sure that those measures will work. A pandemic in which one third of the population falls ill, with waves of outbreaks lasting months, would be far more than a "temporary inconvenience."

But the final flu plan, released earlier this month, is much more dire. It estimates that pandemic deaths in the United States could approach 2 million, more on a par with the 1918 contagion. The plan also talks about the widespread breakdown in municipal services and social order that could occur, including the loss of public transportation and electricity, and food shortages.

Flu experts have criticized the U.S. plan for relying too much on the antiviral drug Tamiflu. No one knows if it would work against a pandemic flu strain, and even in the best-case scenario the United States would have enough for only about 1 in 4 people. A pandemic flu vaccine, another cornerstone of the federal response, wouldn't be widely available until 2010 at the earliest. But the final plan does acknowledge shortcomings: In a pandemic, communities would be on their own, with little or no help from state or federal authorities.

Over the summer, HHS polled 60,000 people and 20,000 doctors and asked them what they knew about avian flu or flu pandemics. The answer: not much. They also asked them what they thought about the department's "priority groups" for handing out a potential pandemic flu vaccine. Respondents were offended by the notion of priorities, even though they agreed that first responders like doctors should be at the head of the line. HHS now calls them "predefined groups."

In the next three months, HHS's Leavitt will travel to communities around the country, urging people to start querying their workplaces or neighborhood schools on how each would handle a pandemic. The risk, Sandman says, is having people turn around five or 10 years from now and say, "Why did you scare us? Why did we spend all this money? This pandemic was no big deal." But, he adds, "it is better to waste time, money, and emotional energy than to risk stumbling into a crisis unwarned and unprepared."

Influenza Economics

By Cinda Becker
Modern Healthcare, November 7, 2005

Influenza, the commonly known name for a sometimes deadly group of ever-mutating viruses, is for the U.S. healthcare industry the annual little nest egg that can boost hospital admissions and potentially nurse a sick balance sheet through a long, bitter winter.

Clinicians say only the most fragile patients—the very young and the very old—are hospitalized for flu, and most frequently they are admitted with complex diagnoses that extend hospital stays and thin margins. Yet when well-managed, there is some profit to be made.

But all bets are off in the event of a pandemic. Experts warn that a virulent avian flu strain in its worst scenario won't discriminate between victims, stretching hospital capacity with normally healthy patients. From a financial standpoint, that could mean a positive bottom line only if a hospital is fully prepared. More likely, hospitals fear, a pandemic will create a surge in admissions that ultimately breaks down an already overstretched and unprepared healthcare system.

With three pandemics in the last century, epidemiologists say the world is overdue for another and the most threatening virus is the so-called avian influenza A virus, also known as H5N1. The virus occurs naturally among birds, but there have been several cases since 1997 in which the virus spread from birds to humans, who have little or no immune protection against it, according to the Centers for Disease Control and Prevention. Cases of human-to-human transmission have been rare, but if the virus were to mutate, the world could have a new and devastating pandemic on its hands.

That would present a stark new challenge for the hospital industry, which has had mixed results in cost-effectively treating influenza year after year. Still, in the winter months, hospital financial experts almost count on an outbreak.

"Influenza is one of the biggest predictors of hospital utilization and occupancy rate. It is the driver in the winter months," said Dale Schumacher, a physician and president of the Rockburn Institute in Baltimore, a health services research and consulting firm. "What we don't know is when the flu season will hit so we can adjust staffing."

In a typical flu year, most influenza patients are chronically ill people "that would otherwise be managed outside the hospital" had they not been bitten by the flu bug, Schumacher said. "Any time you can function at optimal occupancy rates, you ought to be able to put dollars on the bottom line. . . . Whether it leads to profitability depends on the individual hospital capacity and the kinds of patients."

Driving Volume

Publicly traded hospital companies would not explicitly say that their profit margins rely on the coughing, wheezing and fevers of the public, but winter season financial reports frequently note the acuity of the past flu season to justify volumes. For example, in its quarterly financial report in May, Universal Health Services, King of Prussia, Pa., noted revenue growth in its hospital division "resulted primarily from admissions growth and an increase in revenue per adjusted patient day." The admission growth was attributed in part to "a busier flu season."

Similarly, last February, HCA reported in its quarterly financial report that a strong fourth-quarter flu season in 2003 raised the bar for admissions growth in the fourth quarter of 2004, when flu-related or pulmonary admissions decreased by approximately 18.3%. Emergency room visits decreased 5.4% during the fourth quarter of 2004 from the year-ago period, "primarily due to higher flu-related volumes during the fourth quarter of 2003," while flu-related or pulmonary emergency room visits declined by approximately 31.7%, HCA reported.

"The biggest thing flu does is make volume numbers go up," said Frank Morgan, a research analyst for investment banking firm Jefferies & Co. Typically falling in the fourth quarter and sometimes stretching into the first quarter of the new calendar year, flu season is not necessarily a huge profit-maker, he said. A labor-intensive medical condition, reimbursement for this tends to be lower than it would be for high-margin services like surgery. Although the profits are smaller, treating flu patients is not generally money-losing and "stocks seem to react at least in the short term to whatever the level of flu season is," Morgan said.

In 2003, hospitals nationwide discharged 54,944 flu patients who stayed an average 3.5 days, according to the Agency for Healthcare Research and Quality. The majority of those patients—nearly 60%—were admitted from hospital emergency rooms. That compares with the 1.3 million pneumonia patients who were discharged from hospitals the same year, staying an average 5.7 days and totaling up aggregate charges of $26 billion. More than 70% of those patients were admitted from hospital emergency departments.

More recently, in the year ended September 30, 2004, 24,679 Medicare patients were discharged from hospitals nationwide with a principal diagnosis of influenza, according to Solucient, a healthcare business information company. Those patients stayed an average 5.3 days, racking up charges of over $15,000 per case. The hospital was reimbursed on average $4,300 per case, but the average cost per case was a little over $6,500—a negative margin.

Also, in terms of cost, in the year ended March 1, there were 8,816 cases of influenza combined with other diagnoses and 5,182 cases of influenza alone at 370 hospitals in Premier's hospital alliance Perspective database. The average length of stay for the more complex flu cases was 5.3 days with an average cost per case of $7,420.32, according to Premier. When influenza was the only diagnosis, patients stayed an

> No one seems to be asking whether an avian flu pandemic will be profitable for healthcare providers.

average 4.3 days at an average cost per case of $5,383.33.

No one seems to be asking whether an avian flu pandemic will be profitable for healthcare providers, but then not many hospitals are asking themselves if garden variety influenza is a money-losing or profit-making proposition as it stands.

"We haven't taken a look at the book of business on flu," said Teri D'Agostino, a spokeswoman for the University of Rochester (N.Y.) Medical Center. "The reason is it's kind of a secondary diagnosis. Most of the time they are older patients with chronic underlying conditions." Rochester is one of four medical sites nationwide where the National Institute of Allergy and Infectious Diseases is testing the safety of an experimental avian flu vaccine manufactured by Sanofi Pasteur on 450 healthy people between the ages of 18 and 64. Vanderbilt University Medical Center, Nashville, Tenn., another participant, administered its first vaccine on Nov. 1 to a physician.

The Tipping Point

A bad bout of flu can be the tipping point that robs such patients of their last vestiges of independent living, sending them to the hospital and then a nursing home. Waiting for available beds at a nursing home inevitably extends the length of a hospital stay, racking up more costs, she said. Rochester officials know that medical patients tend to stay longer than surgical patients—8.3 days for medical patients versus 7.9 days for surgical. Meanwhile, reimbursement for medical patients on average is just half the amount for surgical patients, D'Agostino said. "I would call it a thinner margin and in extreme cases, it certainly is money-losing," she said. In the winter months, the hospital assumes there will be a higher number of patient days, so "staffing does flex up . . . and this is undoubtedly contributed to by the flu," D'Agostino said.

At Crozer-Keystone Health System, Springfield, Pa., where Schumacher consults, respiratory distress seems to be the diagnostic group that spikes during flu season. Such patients flood the system's four hospital sites, doctor offices and emergency rooms, said Kathy Scullin, a Crozer-Keystone spokeswoman. One day in December 2004, inpatient admissions jumped from 700 to 825 patients systemwide. "In our health system, we look at it as a strain on our resources," Scullin said. "Flu puts stresses on our system, and it's difficult to anticipate that."

Dire Predictions

In 1999, researchers at the CDC investigated the potential economic impact of pandemic influenza in the U.S. That study by Martin Meltzer, Nancy Cox and Keiji Fukuda projected that in 1995 dollars, hospitalization of patients 65 years and older would cost a mean $6,856 per case plus or minus $3,200—a great deal of variability as there always is in hospital care, Meltzer said. The average outpatient visit for the same segment of the population would be an average $102 plus or minus $60, according to the study.

The authors estimated that the next influenza pandemic would cause as many as 207,000 deaths, as many as 734,000 hospitalizations, and up to 42 million outpatient visits. The estimated economic impact would be as much as $166.5 billion, excluding commercial and societal costs, the authors said.

According to HHS' Pandemic Influenza Plan released last week, the annual flu season in the U.S. results on average in 36,000 deaths, 226,000 hospitalizations and between $1 billion and $3 billion in direct medical costs—much of the impact because of secondary complications such as pneumonia and heart problems. In projecting the impact of a pandemic, HHS extrapolated data from the severe pandemic of 1918 and the moderate pandemics of 1958 and 1968. Based on the assumption that 30% of the population will fall ill, HHS projected that a moderate pandemic would generate 865,000 hospitalizations and a severe pandemic, 9.9 million hospitalizations. Under both scenarios, half the infected population—45 million—would require outpatient medical care.

Approximately $6.1 billion of $7.1 billion in federal money promised to fuel the national strategy against avian flu was earmarked for vaccine development, production and stockpiling, as an effective and timely vaccine is widely considered the best weapon against the scourge.

In 2000, Highmark Blue Cross and Blue Shield in Pittsburgh studied 186,000 of its members enrolled in its Medicare HMO product to see if it was cost-effective for the health plan to give flu shots away, said Denise Grabner, a Highmark spokeswoman. The analysis found that members who were vaccinated against flu saved the plan 15%, or $54, in costs every month.

The federal allocation for vaccine development would represent "a huge boost for novel production techniques" as well as for technologies to screen for and identify flu outbreaks, said Geoffrey Porges, senior biotech analyst for Sanford Bernstein, an institutional equity research firm. That kind of money "is not going to make or break any pharmaceutical company," Porges said. The market for flu antivirals is about $1.5 billion worldwide with the bulk of that being Roche's Tamiflu, he said. Flu vaccines constitute an estimated $1.3

billion worldwide market. That's not much in the pharmaceutical world; the $2.5 billion worldwide market for influenza preventives and treatments is equal to just one-fifth of the market for cholesterol-lowering drugs, Porges noted.

Three Things You Don't Know About AIDS in Africa

By Emily Oster
Esquire, December 1, 2006

*At just twenty-six, economist Emily Oster may have the highest controver-
sies-generated-to-years-in-academia ratio of anyone in her field. That's
because, as a Ph.D. student at Harvard, she chose to hop the fence and
explore a topic already claimed by doctors, social scientists, and policy
wonks: the AIDS epidemic in Africa. Her studies suggest some uncomfortable possibilities—not least that the so-called experts have gotten their
approach to the crisis dead wrong.*

*Now a Becker Fellow at the University of Chicago, Oster continues to blur
academic boundaries with further work on AIDS and a volatile new interest: the reported wave of female infanticide in Asia.*

When I began studying the HIV epidemic in Africa a few years
ago, there were few other economists working on the topic and
almost none on the specific issues that interested me. It's not that
the questions I wanted to answer weren't being asked. They were.
But they were being asked by anthropologists, sociologists, and public-health officials.

That's an important distinction. These disciplines believe that cultural differences—differences in how entire groups of people think
and act—account for broader social and regional trends. AIDS
became a disaster in Africa, the thinking goes, because Africans
didn't know how to deal with it.

Economists like me don't trust that argument. We assume everyone is fundamentally alike; we believe circumstances, not culture,
drive people's decisions, including decisions about sex and disease.

I've studied the epidemic from that perspective. I'm one of the few
people who have done so. And I've learned that a lot of what we've
been told about it is wrong. Below are three things the world needs
to know about AIDS in Africa.

1) It's the wrong disease to attack.

Approximately 6 percent of adults in sub-Saharan Africa are
infected with HIV; in the United States, the number is around 0.8
percent. Very often, this disparity is attributed to differences in sexual behavior—in the number of sexual partners, the types of sexual

---

activities, and so on. But these differences cannot, in fact, be seen in the data on sexual behavior. So what actually accounts for the gulf in infection rates?

According to my research, the major difference lies in transmission rates of the virus. For a given unprotected sexual relationship with an HIV-infected person, Africans are between four and five times more likely than Americans to become infected with HIV themselves. This stark fact accounts for virtually all of the difference in population-wide HIV rates in the two regions.

There is more than one reason why HIV spreads more easily in Africa than America, but the most important one seems to be related to the prevalence of other sexually transmitted infections. Estimates suggest that around 11 percent of individuals in Africa have untreated bacterial sexually transmitted infections at any given time and close to half have the herpes virus. Because many of these infections cause open sores on the genitals, transmission of the HIV virus is much more efficient.

How much people care about dying from AIDS ten years from now depends on how many years they expect to live today and how enjoyable they expect those future years to be.

So what do we learn from this? First, the fact that Africa is so heavily affected by HIV has very little to do with differences in sexual behavior and very much to do with differences in circumstances. Second, and perhaps more important, there is potential for significant reductions in HIV transmission in Africa through the treatment of other sexually transmitted diseases. Such an approach would cost around $3.50 per year per life saved. Treating AIDS itself costs around $300 per year. There are reasons to provide AIDS treatment in Africa, but cost-effectiveness is not one of them.

2) It won't disappear until poverty does.

In the United States, the discovery of the HIV epidemic led to dramatic changes in sexual behavior. In Africa, it didn't. Yet in both places, encouraging safe sexual behavior has long been standard practice. Why haven't the lessons caught on in Africa?

The key is to think about *why* we expect people to change their behavior in response to HIV—namely because, in a world with HIV, sex carries a larger risk of death than it does in a world without HIV. But how much people care about dying from AIDS ten years from now depends on how many years they expect to live today and how enjoyable they expect those future years to be.

My studies show that while there have been very limited changes in sexual behavior in Africa *on average*, Africans who are richer or who live in areas with higher life expectancies have changed their behavior more. And men in Africa have responded in almost exactly the same way to their relative "life forecasts" as gay men in the United States did in the 1980s. To put it bluntly, if income and life expectancy in Africa were the same as they are in the United States, we would see the same change in sexual behavior—and the AIDS epidemic would begin to slow.

3) There is less of it than we thought—but it's spreading as fast as ever.

According to the UN, the HIV rates in Botswana and Zimbabwe are around 30 percent, and it's more than 10 percent in many other countries. These estimates are relied on by policymakers, researchers, and the popular press. Yet many people who study the AIDS epidemic believe that the numbers are inflated.

The reason is quite simple: bias in who is tested. The UN's estimates are *not* based on diagnoses of whole populations or even a random sample. They are based on tests of pregnant women at prenatal clinics. And in Africa, sexually active women of childbearing age have the highest rates of HIV infection.

To eliminate the bias, I took a new approach to estimating the HIV infection rate: I inferred it from mortality data. The idea is simple: In a world without HIV, we have some expectation of what the death rate will be. In a world with HIV, we observe the actual death rate to be higher. The difference between the two gives an estimate of the number of people who have died from AIDS, and we can use that figure to estimate the prevalence of HIV in the population.

My work suggests that the HIV rates reported by the UN are about three times too high. Which sounds like good news—but isn't. The overall number of HIV-positive people may be lower than we thought, but my study, which estimated changes in the infection rate over time, also drew a second, chilling conclusion: In Africa, HIV is spreading as quickly as ever.

The HIV Trade-Off

By David Batstone
Sojourners, February 2006

Karl Barth's prescription for an engaged Christian is often quoted: Keep in one hand the Bible and in the other hand the daily newspaper. I tweak the advice of the famed Swiss theologian for my own discipline and keep in my newspaper hand copies of two highly regarded dailies: *The Wall Street Journal* and *The New York Times*. Most folks read the news that reinforces their own point of view. Absorbing a steady diet of adversarial positions and the statistics that accompany them helps us to identify those idols closest to home.

That's also why I keep up a subscription to *Forbes*, the magazine that proudly touts itself as a publication for "the world's business leaders." I was leafing through a copy of *Forbes* recently, and an article caught my eye: "Treating HIV Doesn't Pay." The tagline was equally jarring: "It is humane to pay for AIDS drugs in Africa, but it isn't economical. The same dollars spent on prevention would save more lives."

The piece penned by Emily Oster, a graduate student of economics at Harvard, applies an economic cost-benefit analysis to a serious social crisis. She pits pouring resources into antiretroviral therapy that may save individual lives against a preventative strategy that would arrest the spread of the epidemic,

Oster does a yeoman's service by dispelling a widely held myth that AIDS has spread in Africa primarily due to the undisciplined exercise of libido—in simple terms, the idea that Africans have more sex and more sexual partners. While sexual behavior certainly plays into the AIDS epidemic in Africa (as it does everywhere), Oster points out that its transmission can be traced in large part to untreated infections such as gonorrhea and syphilis that create open sores and serve as a hotbed for HIV.

Moving from that assumption, she suggests two measures that would be more effective than treating individuals with HIV. First, shift precious resources to deploy antibiotics to treat sexually transmitted infections that precipitate the spread of HIV. Second, invest in education that will help Africans better understand how HIV spreads and how to act preventatively. Both methods, Oster argues, would be more cost-effective: "Antiretroviral treatment is around

100 times as expensive in preventing AIDS deaths as treating other sexually transmitted infections and around 25 times as expensive as education."

Oster is not cruel. She acknowledges that morality and compassion may compel us to jettison a cost-benefit analysis and opt to treat the afflicted with mercy. But she also helps us understand that we may be trading off compassion for more feasible long-term solutions.

The facile reaction to her dilemma is to pretend that we do not have to make such a trade-off. We can invest in treatment, prevention, and education. Surely she's built a false divide; can't we just integrate all these efforts into a comprehensive strategy?

The truth of the matter is that health organizations do not have unlimited funds at their disposal. It would be right to point out to wealthy nations the shame of this scarcity in a world of plenty. But a prophetic "should be" does not erase the harsh truth of what exists in front of us. The funds available to health agencies are insufficient to address the crisis.

So how do they best address the spread of AIDS in Africa, India, China, and elsewhere? Oster's analysis helps, but it also leaves out some serious considerations. The number of lives saved is not the only goal of intervention. A human society can be torn apart by the loss of an entire generation of parents, educators, and leaders. The future of a society depends on both its young and its old, on vitality and wisdom.

It is an even more intangible objective to promote a spirit of compassion and hope in a society. But it is a sacred mystery we deny at our peril. The gift—and sometimes the curse—of being human is our empathetic impulse. To suppress compassion and turn wholly to calculation would tear out the soul of society.

Unfortunately, we are stuck with a tragic dilemma. Everyone's good dream will break somebody's heart.

Death by Mosquito

By Christine Gorman
Time, July 26, 2004

As current trends make clear, AIDS is surpassing the Black Death as the most devastating plague ever to afflict the human race. That helps explain the sense of desperation that permeated the 15th International Conference on HIV and AIDS in Bangkok last week. But in a cruel irony, all the well-deserved attention paid to AIDS over the past few years has overshadowed the rapid comeback of a second, nearly-as-deadly plague—malaria. The latest figures suggest that malaria sickened 300 million people last year and killed 3 million—most of them under age 5. (AIDS last year killed just over 3 million people.) What makes the malaria deaths particularly tragic is that malaria, unlike AIDS, can be cured.

Countries in sub-Saharan Africa have suffered the brunt of this renewed assault, but nations in temperate zones, including the U.S., are not immune. A malaria outbreak in Florida last summer that hospitalized seven people was the first extended case of local transmission on U.S. soil in nearly 20 years. The cause was almost certainly a parasite that hopped a ride in a human or a mosquito on an international flight or ocean vessel, since none of the patients had recently ventured overseas.

Despite these setbacks, there is reason for hope. Doctors have made remarkable progress over the past few years in the treatment of drug-resistant malaria by combining several compounds—the most powerful of which is derived from an ancient Chinese herbal remedy that cures 90% of patients in three days. Meanwhile, community groups, nonprofit organizations and governments are redoubling efforts to control the mosquitoes that cause the disease through the sale and distribution of insecticide-treated bed nets and the indoor spraying of antimosquito pesticides. And after a few notably fiery fits and starts, there appears to be a real consensus among health officials about how to proceed. Certainly, the need for action has never been clearer.

Doctors have long suspected that the malaria problem was getting worse, but the most searing proof has come to light in just the past year. Researchers believe the average number of cases of malaria per year in Africa has quadrupled since the 1980s. A study in the journal Lancet last June reported that the death rate due to malaria has at least doubled among children in eastern and southern Africa;

some rural areas have seen a heartbreaking 11-fold jump in mortality. "The death rates from malaria are as high as those from HIV," says Dr. Christa Hook, coordinator of the malaria working group for Doctors Without Borders. "In many ways, it's a kind of silent Holocaust."

> "The death rates from malaria are as high as those from HIV. In many ways, it's a kind of silent Holocaust."—Dr. Christa Hook, Doctors Without Borders

Recognition of malaria's toll on the global economy is growing. Economist Jeffrey Sachs, director of Columbia University's Earth Institute, estimates that countries hit hardest by the most severe form of malaria have annual economic growth rates 1.3 percentage points lower than those in which malaria is not a serious problem. Sachs points out that the economies of Greece, Portugal and Spain expanded rapidly only after malaria was eradicated in those countries in the 1950s. In other words, fighting malaria is good for business—as many companies with overseas operations have long understood. By the end of this year, Exxon Mobil, which plans to expand activities in the sub-Saharan countries of Chad, Cameroon, Angola, Equatorial Guinea and Nigeria, hopes to triple its funding for antimalaria projects and research, from $2 million to $6 million. But the malaria problem is bigger than Exxon Mobil or even Bill and Melinda Gates. Government action is needed.

To better understand why malaria has become such a threat and what can be done to stop the disease, it helps to know a little biology. Malaria is caused by four closely related parasites, the deadliest of which is Plasmodium falciparum, which has a particular fondness for anopheles mosquitoes. The parasites enter the bloodstream when an infected mosquito bites a human. Then they multiply inside the host's liver and red blood cells. (That's why pregnant women, who make lots of blood to nourish their growing fetus, are especially vulnerable.) Eventually the red blood cells burst with a new generation of parasites, causing fever, shivering, pain and sometimes death. The cycle of transmission is complete when another mosquito bites an infected person and picks up more parasites.

You might expect that one bout of malaria would lead to lifelong protection against the disease. But for complicated reasons, that is not the case. The illness tends to be less severe in adults who are continually exposed to the parasites. But when young children become infected, they are much more likely to suffer severe anemia and convulsions that may lead to permanent brain damage and death.

For decades, the best treatment for malaria was an inexpensive medication called chloroquine, first discovered in Germany in 1934 by a researcher working for Bayer. Chloroquine was so effective that it seemed it might vanquish malaria forever. But by the 1970s, the drug had been used so widely to treat all kinds of fevers, not just those caused by malaria, that the malaria parasites became resistant and doctors had to turn to a second medication, called sulfadoxine-pyrimethamine, or SP. But within five years, the parasites started to develop resistance to SP as well. Today resistance to both drugs is rampant in many parts of Africa, where resistant malaria parasites are the leading cause of death.

> To be successful, any antimalaria campaign must do two things: treat the illness and prevent the transmission of parasites.

At the same time, efforts to control anopheles mosquitoes have been more or less abandoned. Part of the problem was the realization that malaria could never be completely eradicated from tropical regions the way it had been in the U.S. and other countries in temperate zones. There was also a growing backlash against DDT, a pesticide that is highly effective at attacking mosquitoes but whose indiscriminate use in agriculture killed many fish, beneficial insects and birds. Although only small amounts of DDT are needed to control malaria—usually in indoor-spraying campaigns—its toxic reputation made cash-strapped governments in Africa, which often must rely heavily on international donors, hesitant to use it.

So much for how things got so bad. The silver lining to all this heartache is that the outlines of a workable solution have at long last emerged. No one is promising an end to all deaths from malaria. But doctors estimate that hundreds of millions of people could be spared the illness and the mortality rate could be cut in half. The catch: although astonishingly inexpensive (at least by the industrial world's standards), an effective response is still beyond the financial resources of the poorest nations of the world, particularly those in Africa. There simply can be no progress without help from the developed world.

To be successful, any antimalaria campaign must do two things: treat the illness and prevent the transmission of parasites. Several pilot studies conducted in Africa have proved that combination therapy, in which at least one of the medications is derived from a plant called Artemisia annua, or sweet wormwood, easily destroys drug-resistant malarial parasites in the bloodstream. Using several drugs at once, often in the same pill, greatly decreases the risk that the parasites will become resistant. As an added bonus, artemisinin, the active ingredient in Artemisia annua, acts very quickly, further decreasing the chances of drug resistance.

The full three-day course of treatment with artemisinin-based combination therapy costs from $1 to $10 a person, depending on whether it is purchased in the public or private sector. Unfortunately, that's at least 10 times the price of current, albeit ineffective, treatment programs. Most impoverished African governments simply cannot afford to foot the entire bill for combination therapy and the training required to give it, and the same holds true for the majority of their private citizens, many of whom already spend a third of their income on malaria treatment.

Although nearly every developed country and most major international aid organizations have said they are ready to help finance artemisinin-based treatment in Africa, that support has not always been forthcoming. Some health experts believe a report on artemisinin-containing therapy due out from the U.S. Institute of Medicine this week will dissolve any lingering reluctance.

And what about prevention? Many African countries are working to sell or distribute low-cost insecticide-impregnated mosquito nets. These function as traps for mosquitoes, which are attracted by the carbon dioxide that sleepers exhale and are then killed by the insecticide. The nets are portable, so they can be taken along by their owners if they need to move. In villages where at least 80% of pregnant women and children under age 5 sleep beneath insecticide-impregnated mosquito nets, the rate of illness for all residents has dropped dramatically. Unfortunately, only 1% or 2% of people in malarial zones sleep under mosquito nets. Also, most nets need to be retreated every six months, and they are less effective in areas where anopheles mosquitoes bite all day long instead of just at night.

A more controversial but nonetheless effective method of reducing transmission is to spray DDT inside huts and other buildings. Intriguingly, DDT is often better at repelling mosquitoes than killing them. This requires much less pesticide than was once sprayed on crops and swamps. Indeed, if DDT had been used only for medicinal purposes, it might never have acquired its toxic reputation. An international antipesticide treaty that took effect last May makes an exception for the use of DDT in malarial areas, but some health experts are worried that the bureaucratic headache of applying for an exemption will limit the effectiveness of DDT.

Recent experience in South Africa shows just how well DDT can work. In 1996 the South African government, under pressure from international and domestic environmental groups, decided to phase out its use of DDT in residential spraying and rely instead on pesticides containing pyrethroid chemicals. Unfortunately, it turned out that many anopheles mosquitoes in South Africa were resistant to pyrethroids. The number of cases of malaria, which had been hovering between 8,000 and 13,000 a year, grew steadily worse, and by the year 2000 it had reached 64,000 cases, with 423 deaths. When the government reintroduced DDT spraying in the middle of that year, the results were dramatic. The number of cases fell almost immediately. By the end of 2001, when doctors began treating their patients with Coartem, a single, multidrug pill that includes an artemisinin derivative, the number of cases had been cut in half. In 2003 the number of deaths was down to 146.

Even environmentalists had to admit that DDT was necessary. "I wasn't very happy about it, but we are what you'd call pragmatic conservationists," says Gerhard Verdoorn, chairman of South Africa's Endangered Wildlife Trust, which had earlier lobbied the South African government to drop the pesticide and now helps train the 350 or so DDT sprayers who are employed each year. "We can't just look after animals and not care if people die."

That's the kind of attitude that will make a difference in the battle against malaria. The know-how to control the disease already exists. What is not so clear is whether there is the necessary commitment—financial and political—to make it happen.

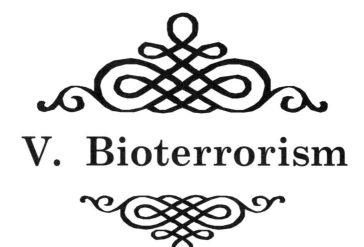

V. Bioterrorism

Editor's Introduction

Soon after the terrorist attacks of September 11, 2001, the American people were traumatized anew, this time by letters laced with anthrax, an infectious and deadly disease, mailed to government officials and news agencies. Since that time government agencies in various countries have mobilized to protect their citizens from bioterrorism, defined here as the deliberate release of biological agents such as bacteria, toxins, or viruses by terrorist operatives with the intention of sickening or killing people, plants, or animals. If effectively weaponized, a biological agent could severely cripple a nation by directly harming its citizens, poisoning its food or water supply, or simply creating a climate of fear that disrupts everyday life.

Biological agents are particularly attractive to terrorists because they are often difficult to detect, have a delayed reaction time, with victims not showing signs of illness for hours or days, and, perhaps most important, possess tremendous psychological power, breeding fear and insecurity to a greater degree than conventional terrorism. Nevertheless, according to the U.S. Centers for Disease Control and Prevention, the effectiveness of a bioterrorist attack varies greatly depending on the agent used. Anthrax, for example, cannot be spread from person to person, while smallpox can quite effectively. Like a naturally occurring epidemic outbreak, a bioterrorist attack would require a particular response from authorities to contain the damage: For instance, medical facilities would need to be set up, victims quarantined, drug treatments prepped, and the general population tested to measure the extent of the exposure. However, unlike with a naturally occurring epidemic, law enforcement officials and intelligence agencies would use forensic testing and surveillance to identify and arrest the perpetrators.

While governments in the post-9/11 world have made concerted efforts to prepare for a biological terrorist attack, some critics have argued that the threat of bioterrorism is overstated, that the unstable nature of biological agents makes them severely limited weapons. On the other hand, some believe that genetic engineering will soon make bioterrorism a far more potent threat. Regardless, a biological terrorist attack on a large scale using current technology would, at the very least, create a mass panic, inflicting both a psychological and an economic blow on society. The articles presented in this section offer differing views on bioterrorism as well as the preparations under way to counter such an attack.

In "The Bioterroism Scare," Philip Alcabes, arguing that the threat of bioterrorism is overhyped, presents an overview of the history of biological attacks and a critique of current counter-bioterrorism tactics. The writer of the next piece, "Biological Weapons," counters Alcabes's argument to some degree by suggesting that bioterrorism preparedness is in fact a boon to Third World countries because it funds research into vaccines, leading to potential break-throughs in preventing such diseases as the Marburg and Ebola viruses. Next, Ingrid Wickelgren, in "Pox Unlocked?" weighs the pros and cons of current efforts by researchers to study the smallpox virus, which was virtually wiped out by the World Health Organization (WHO) in the 1970s. In the subsequent article, "Identifying Airborne Pathogens in Time to Respond," Gabriele Rennie discusses new technologies currently in development to monitor for the release of biological agents. Next, Eric Lipton reports on how Project Bio-Shield, a program established by the Bush administration after the 2001 anthrax attacks, has failed to stockpile drugs in the necessary amounts to counteract a serious biological epidemic outbreak.

Finally, Barton Peppert, in "The Biodefense Buildup: Fallout for Other Research Areas," argues that the George W. Bush administration's emphasis on preparing for a bioterrorist attack may actually erode the nation's public health infrastructure by shifting resources away from more immediate—if less spectacular—threats.

The Bioterrorism Scare

BY PHILIP ALCABES
THE AMERICAN SCHOLAR, SPRING 2004

Since the fall of 2001, when America embarked on a "war on ter-rorism" and federal officials started warning us about the next plague, here are some events that have not happened: a U.S. epi-demic of sudden acute respiratory syndrome (SARS), a widespread anthrax outbreak, any smallpox attack, the discovery of hard evi-dence of a biological weapons program in Iraq. Yet the talk about "biopreparedness" continues. Some people in Washington want the Centers for Disease Control and Prevention to be transferred from the Department of Health and Human Services to Homeland Secu-rity. There is even a professional journal, Biosecurity and Bioterror-ism, devoted to learned discussions of the topic. Is it sound public policy to rush to protect the country against the threat of attack with germs that could cause an epidemic? Does the bio in biosecu-rity mean that we should turn our public health into a matter of civil defense? Or have we Americans been sold a bill of goods?

Throughout history, the responses to both actual communicable disease and the threat of it have been guided by the metaphor of the stranger as the spreader of contagion. Allegations that epidemic dis-ease was caused by foreigners are ancient. Thucydides reported that his contemporaries, in the fifth century B.C., attributed the Plague of Athens to Ethiopians. Later on, such thinking was refined to impute causation specifically to enemy foreigners. Many European and American authors still believe that the Black Death entered western Europe after the Mongols, besieging the city of Kefe (or Kaffa, now Feodosiya in Ukraine) in 1346, catapulted into the Euro-pean-held city the corpses of comrades who had died of plague. When the siege was lifted, the theory goes, the disease reached Genoa aboard ships. Although Kefe clearly experienced plague in 1346, the story of its source is almost certainly apocryphal: Xenop-sylla cheopis, the flea that usually carries the plague bacillus, has affinity only for warm bodies and will desert a corpse within hours of death. But the myth's persistence attests to the readiness of some, even centuries later, to believe that epidemics were caused by enemies.

Similarly, Londoners believed that the Great Plague of 1665 was brought by the Dutch, with whom England was then at war (echoes of that belief appear in both Defoe's Journal of the Plague Year and

Samuel Pepys's Diary), although there is no evidence that plague in fact came to England from Holland. The great influenza pandemic of 1918–19, which killed more than 20 million people—possibly as many as 40 million—in a world at war, was attributed to various enemies. In fact, the name by which we remember this epidemic, "Spanish Flu," seems to have been a compromise acceptable to the warring parties (Spain was neutral in the war). And in a telling instance, very shortly after Germany broke its pact with the Soviet Union and invaded its former ally, Hitler used the term Pestherd—"plague focus"—to refer to Russia, accusing the Soviets of infecting Europe with Jewish "bacilli." It was the metaphor of foreign culpability for disease turned inside out, Hitler imputing pathogenic properties to Jews and creating a new enemy by alleging that it was Russia that had spawned them. More recently, Tanzanians attributed the high death rate from AIDS in their Kagera province to HIV infections brought by Idi Amin's Ugandan troops, who crossed the border into Tanzania in the late 1970s. "It made sense, then," Laurie Garrett writes in The Coming Plague, "to assume that the new disease came from old enemies." When West Nile encephalitis made its Western hemisphere debut in New York in 1999, epidemiologists received calls from the FBI; they (and the CIA, too) were concerned that it might be the work of foreign bioterrorists.

> The Stranger Spreading Germs shows up often in literature and film.

The Stranger Spreading Germs shows up often in literature and film. Alessandro Manzoni's 1821 novel, I Promessi Sposi, attributes the advance of plague in 1629 to the German army, then campaigning through the valleys of northern Italy in the Thirty Years' War. In the novel, foreigners, particularly the French, come under suspicion in plague-ridden Milan, where they are accused of "daubing" plague-inducing substances on walls or sprinkling plague powders on the streets; those found guilty of such felonious behavior are tortured to death. In F. W. Murnau's classic silent film Nosferatu, plague arrives in Bremen by sea, brought from the East by the odious Other, the undead Nosferatu. In 1922, just after the carnage of World War I and the far greater mortality of the Spanish Flu pandemic, Murnau depicted Evil as the man who was beyond death, the inscrutable and indomitable being who brings pestilence from the benighted Ausland.

Sometimes, of course, epidemics have come from the enemy foreigner. Clearly, Cortés was able to conquer Mexico because of smallpox. The disease appeared among the Taino on Hispaniola in 1518, brought by Spaniards who had colonized the island; later, it would contribute to the Taino's extinction. By 1519 smallpox was in Cuba. Cortés, who was secretary to the governor of Cuba, left to take Tenochtitlán from the Aztec chief relief expedition against the Aztecs after they repulsed Cortés's initial sallies, brought smallpox to the Aztecs. The disease, to which the Aztecs were immunologically naïve, so diminished their numbers that Cortés had only to finish them off. Smallpox thence spread southeward, killing the Incan emperor Huayna Capac and then his son in 1524–25, and plunging their people into civil war. Francisco Pizarro had little more to do to vanquish the Incas than march into Cuzco.

> In the French and Indian War, in the early 1760s, smallpox does seem to have been spread deliberately.

It is unlikely that the Spaniards infected the American natives deliberately—and the Aztecs, at least, seemed to interpret the devastation as evidence of divine disfavor, not treachery on the part of Spain. But in the French and Indian War, in the early 1760s, smallpox does seem to have been spread deliberately. During the conflict known as Pontiac's Rebellion, Sir Jeffrey Amherst, the British commanding general, approved a plan to distribute smallpox-contaminated blankets "to innoculate the Indians" besieging Fort Pitt, at the fork of the Ohio River. That epidemic smallpox occurred in the Ohio Valley at the time is an established fact.

Around the same time, the Polish army considered producing cannon shells filled with the saliva of rabid dogs, in an attempt to poison the air the enemy breathed. Later, during World War I, the German biological warfare program sought to create animal epidemics—epizootics, in the lingo of epidemiology—that would diminish their enemies' ability to fight. German agents deliberately infected their neutral trading partners' livestock and animal feed with the agents of glanders (principally an equine disease) and anthrax. Romanian sheep were infected with both microbes in 1916 before export to Russia; more than two hundred Argentine mules intended as dray animals for Allied forces died after being inoculated with both bacteria; French cavalry horses were infected with glanders; and attempts were made to contaminate animal feed in the United States. During World War II, the Third Reich avowedly eschewed use of biological warfare, but one report holds that Colorado beetles were dropped by German airplanes on potato crops in southern England. The U.S. Army claims that the retreating Wehrmacht contaminated a reservoir in Bohemia with sewage, presumably to produce disease in the advancing Soviet army.

The best documented, and most successful, deliberately caused human epidemic was set by the infamous Unit 731 of the Japanese Imperial Army, stationed in conquered China during World War II. In addition to numerous heinous medical "experiments"—tortures, really—the unit dropped plague-carrying fleas on eleven Chinese towns. The number of Chinese who died of plague was probably about seven hundred. Unit 731 also produced cholera. In fact, Japanese soldiers, whom the unit had failed to warn or prepare, died in large numbers after entering Chinese areas seeded with Vibrio cholerae. Some historians put the total number of deaths attributable to the unit's intentional contaminations, including others involving anthrax and typhoid, in the thousands.

In connection with humans deliberately causing epidemics, the smallpox germ, variola virus, is the one we hear most about. It enjoyed a five-hundred-year career as a natural epidemic pathogen, from roughly the late fifteenth century until the late twentieth. Then smallpox was eradicated from the earth. Variola killed several hundred million people in the first half of the twentieth century alone—a public-health menace to be reckoned with. No doubt because of its fearsome reputation, it is the subject of a great number of speculative scenarios about how it might be resurrected as an epidemic scourge.

In fact, though, none of those scenarios is even remotely likely. First, not many people have access to viable smallpox stocks. Second, the disease that variola virus produces is fairly easy to diagnose. Third, vaccination will prevent disease even in already-infected contacts of smallpox cases, and vaccine stocks are reasonably large nowadays. The hubbub about smallpox has had the effect of sharpening physicians' diagnostic skills (indeed, so much so that instances of overdiagnosis produce false alarms) and expanding the supply of available vaccine. At this point, standard public-health procedures, including case diagnosis, contact investigation, and immunization of possibly infected individuals, would be adequate to prevent an outbreak in the unlikely event that some individuals were deliberately infected.

Anthrax is the second most popular topic of bioterrorism conversation. We have seen intentional anthrax infection—the much-ballyhooed postal anthrax events that took place in the fall of 2001. Three characteristics of that outbreak are of note: very few people became ill; very, very few died; and it was almost certainly not produced by a stranger.

Environmental studies in mailrooms indicated that many hundreds of people were probably exposed to anthrax spores that fall, yet only twenty-two people got sick. And of those twenty-two, half had cutaneous anthrax, the rarely-life-threatening skin form of the disease. Only five died. In the jargon of epidemiology, anthrax turned out to be neither very infectious nor very pathogenic. That experience should tell us that spraying anthrax spores from crop dusters or releasing them from aerosol cans into the subway is highly unlikely to make many people ill.

Speculation about subway attacks stems from a real event in March 1995, when the Japanese religious cult Aum Shinrikyo released the nerve toxin sarin in the Tokyo subway system. Twelve people died. Two subsequent attempts to release toxins in the Tokyo subways were foiled. Note that Aum was using a gas, which does not have to be sprayed; it diffuses by itself. This is not how germs are disseminated, and it is a distinction worth bearing in mind. And even that ignores the more central question of likelihood. Large-scale poisonings are not easy to carry out well.

The light death toll from mailed anthrax was a result of the low pathogenicity of the bacteria—half the cases were not pulmonary and were therefore unlikely to be fatal—and the comparative treatability of anthrax disease once detected. Do five deaths constitute a public-health crisis? Along with his colleagues, Victor Sidel, Distinguished Professor of Social Medicine at Albert Einstein College of Medicine in New York, has noted that a fraction of our nation's expenditure on biopreparedness would pay for effective treatment of tuberculosis for all of the two million people who get TB each year in India, thereby preventing close to half a million deaths a year. Half a million deaths because commonly available antibiotics are not affordable—now there's a public-health problem.

The other microbe that is on the lists of virtually all the bioterrorism watchers is the plague bacillus. It is true that Unit 731 produced plague outbreaks in China by dropping infected fleas on towns. But at that time plague was a recurring problem in Asia: a

---

The other microbe that is on the lists of virtually all the bioterrorism watchers is the plague bacillus.

---

ferocious epidemic struck Manchuria in 1910, and another occurred in 1921. (It still is a problem: a large outbreak caused many deaths in India as recently as 1994.) By contrast, despite the presence of Yersinia pestis, the plague bacterium, in wild rodents in the Western Hemisphere, there has never been an extensive epidemic of human plague in this country. Even when plague epidemics moved out of Asia through much of South America, circa 1900, the U.S. saw only a small outbreak in San Francisco's Chinatown. The reason is not that Americans are immune to plague; it is that the urban arrangements that we have been accustomed to for the past two hundred years are inhospitable to the rat-flea-bacillus ecosystem. Such reforms as garbage removal, pest control, and better housing explain why plague disappeared from eastern Europe in the early 1700s and has never troubled as seriously here. Since epidemics of plague are unlikely, should we then worry that terrorists will produce isolated cases? Perhaps, but garden-variety antibiotics are very effective at treating the disease and interrupting transmission. There is no potential for the next catastrophe there.

Other pathogens have been mentioned as possible bioweapons— for example, the agents of tularemia, botulism, and Q fever. These organisms are not generally transmitted from person to person, so they carry little or no outbreak potential. Hemorrhagic fever viruses are sometimes transmitted by mosquitoes or by the bite of infected animals. It has never been shown that they can be manipulated into transportable weapons and then elude standard mosquito- and animal-control programs.

All in all, there is little evidence that terrorists are more likely, or better able, to use microbes as part of their armamentarium than ever before. If there were evidence, would editorialists in the nation's most prestigious medical journal need to argue, as they did in the context of the purported smallpox threat, that public-health decisions should rely on "theoretical data"? Consider the ratio of known success to attempts at bioterrorism.

Jessica Stern reports in The Ultimate Terrorists that the Aum Shinrikyo cult drove three trucks set up to spray botulinum toxin through Tokyo in 1990, but no cases of botulism resulted. Judith Miller, William Broad, and Stephen Engelberg report in their book, Germs, that Aum sprayed anthrax spores from the roof of its building in Tokyo in 1993. This apparently killed some birds, but no humans got sick. Aum members also reportedly tried to procure Ebola virus in the 1990s from what was then Zaire, but if they were able to get the virus, they were unable to produce any cases of Ebola.

> There is little evidence that terrorists are more likely, or better able, to use microbes as part of their armamentarium than ever before.

In the 1960s, a Japanese researcher purposely contaminated food with Salmonella typhi, producing outbreaks of typhoid fever and dysentery, but no deaths. In 1970, four Canadian students got sick after eating food that had been deliberately contaminated with pig ringworm ova. A neo-Nazi group in the U.S. stockpiled the typhoid bacterium in 1972, with the intent of contaminating the water supplies of midwestern cities. They failed. In 1984, members of the Rajneeshee cult contaminated ten Oregon salad bars with Salmonella typhimurium, which causes diarrhea. Federal investigators located 751 cases of salmonellosis, but no deaths occurred. In 1996, twelve people in Texas developed dysentery after eating doughnuts or muffins purposely contaminated with shigella bacteria by a disgruntled lab worker. Again, no deaths.

Presumably, these initiatives represent only a small subset—the known ones—of all attempts to cause mayhem by deliberately introducing germs into a population. Indeed, one systematic study uncovered twenty-nine such attempts to use germs to harm others, although a large proportion seemed to have been perpetrated by single individuals whose aims were against other individuals rather than the population. No doubt there are still more instances, unknown because they were unsuccessful. And yet we can enumerate on the fingers of one hand the deadly epidemics that have in fact been caused deliberately. In the creation of epidemics, the gap between intention and the deed itself is a wide one.

Americans began looking at new infectious diseases as a grave social menace in the early 1990s, and that anxiety resonated loudly after the publication of Laurie Garrett's Coming Plague in 1994. In a sense, the relatively recent worry about bioterrorism is a spin-off of the past decade's concern about the "coming plague." In reality, the intensity of even naturally occurring new epidemics never matches that anticipation.

Our most recent experience with so-called emerging infections has been SARS. It appeared suddenly in southern China in late 2002, the causative virus probably having entered the human population through people who had substantial contact with domestic animals. Although SARS affected more than 8,000 people worldwide and killed more than 700, it was a negligible problem in the U.S. (eight cases, no deaths) and produced no more than a mild epidemic in most other countries: despite the high case-fatality ratio (people diagnosed with SARS had about one chance in ten of dying from the disease), only in China, Hong Kong, Singapore, and Canada were there more than five SARS deaths. Only nineteen countries saw more than a single SARS case. In all the affected areas, the outbreak was brought under control within about six months of its onset.

Two aspects of the SARS experience are important. First, though it is easy to acquire the virus by inhaling respiratory secretions from a SARS sufferer, it also turns out to be easy to prevent or control an outbreak. The key is to use standard infectious-disease-control measures, including case finding and reporting, active surveillance at points of entry to the country, isolation of possible cases, and recommendations against travel to heavily affected regions. None of these measures requires cutting-edge technology; all have been used in controlling communicable disease for well over a century.

Second, SARS made news partly because it was not the expected epidemic. For six months before the advent of SARS, Americans had been worrying very publicly about smallpox. Urged toward apprehension by the federal government, we had alarmed ourselves about the possibility that the long-defunct disease would be reborn in the hands of bioterrorists. The administration made ready, in mid-2002, to vaccinate half a million armed services personnel and half a million health-care workers. The former plan it came close to accomplishing; the latter was abandoned because so many health-care workers refused to show up for vaccination. All of it repeatedly made the headlines and the evening news reports. Yet what happened in the end was not smallpox, or smallpox prevention; it was SARS. Had our faces not already been turned toward epidemic disease and our anxieties about infection elevated, had the news hours not been hungry for new news after a month of relentless coverage of the Iraq war, SARS might not have made such big headlines.

The lesson we should learn from our experience with SARS is that if we are vigilant about spotting new disease outbreaks and equally vigilant about applying public-health programs to curtail their spread, we can limit them, although we cannot ward them off completely. We cannot make life risk-free. Had we dealt with AIDS and West Nile encephalitis the way we dealt with SARS (which, of course, may return in the future and therefore requires continued vigilance), their course might have been different. West Nile, ending only its fifth season in the U.S. as I write, is already virtually a national epidemic; AIDS went national within six or seven years of its appearance. But in its initial season, 1999, in New York City, West Nile virus caused forty-six cases of encephalitis and seven deaths: not negligible, but a public-health problem more minor than Lyme disease (and far less extensive, in New York, than asthma or lead poisoning). AIDS began with a handful of cases—there were only a few hundred in 1981, the first year it was recognized—and the U.S. might have kept the toll fairly small had we had the political nerve to do something about it at the time. The point is that, at the outset, none of these "plagues" were cataclysmic. Epidemics do not work that way. Errant microbes do not find their way into the human ecosystem and wipe out most of the population unannounced. The Andromeda Strain is fantasy.

> The crystal ball with which we divine epidemic mayhem is no clearer now than it used to be.

The crystal ball with which we divine epidemic mayhem is no clearer now than it used to be, and no clearer than the vision with which we try to foresee the coming plague. No one can dispute, after the events of September 11, 2001, that some people wish us harm. However, that harm is not likely to come from bioterrorism. To worry that the Middle Easterner, the Arab, or any Muslim—however the Stranger is configured—will use germs to attack us would be to pretend that we can indeed foresee great epidemics. For two reasons, that is certainly not the case.

First, humans, even ill-tempered and badly behaved humans, have never been able to use germs or weapons to the terrible degree of mortal effect that nature always has been able to use germs. Just four communicable diseases—malaria, smallpox, AIDS, and tuberculosis—killed well over half a billion people in the twentieth century, or about ten times the combined tolls of World Wars I and II, history's bloodiest conflicts. Even today, with good vaccines and effective antibiotics to stop them, infectious diseases kill about 10 million people each year.

The worst catastrophes the world has seen have been not the genocides, however gruesome, but the cataclysmic disease outbreaks. When a few million people are killed by design with Zyklon B, the machete, or the machine gun, it is a horror and an outrage; it shakes our moral faith. But the Black Death killed a third of Europe's population in just four years in the mid-1300s. Smallpox wiped out entire tribes of American natives after Europeans arrived in the 1500s. Plague killed over 50,000 in Moscow alone in just a few months in 1771. The Spanish Flu killed between 20 and 40 million in sixteen months in 1918–19.

And that suddenness is the second point. Prevision is of little help against epidemic disasters. Each of the disasters I just mentioned, and every other great epidemic of history, was unimaginable until the moment it began. But neither is prescience necessary: each epidemic, even the ones that turned out to be most terrible, began slowly, percolated a while,

> It is usually social circumstances that make epidemics possible.

and could have been stopped with conventional public-health responses had anyone acted in time. SARS reminded us of that.

Whether or not the Stranger is an enemy avowedly bent on terror, casting him in the role of microbial evildoer has the perilous effect of distracting us from realizing two truths: the disheartening one that the epidemic crystal ball is always cloudy, and the uncomfortable one that it is usually social circumstances that make epidemics possible and public-health funding that stops them.

Worrying about the germ-bearing Stranger, we forgo the upkeep of a workaday public-health apparatus in favor of fabricating modern wonders. The CDC now operates what it calls a "war room." From there, it can coordinate activities around SARS, West Nile virus, and other infections, as well as bioterrorism—if it can be found—using high-tech communications equipment. The war room is in an "undisclosed location." Once, CDC officials knew they were running a public-health agency. Now, apparently, they must act as if they are in charge of national defense.

After the U.S. Department of Health and Human Services scotched the 2002 plan to vaccinate health-care workers, the CDC announced it would continue its effort to vaccinate police officers and firefighters, despite numerous reasons to stop: several deaths directly attributable to the vaccine; several more possibly attributable; evidence that people who might be predisposed to heart disease (something like 10 or 15 percent of the middleaged population) can be harmed by the vaccination; certainty that people with HIV infection (a sizable percentage of the adult population in some big-city neighborhoods) must not be vaccinated; and of course the complete absence of natural smallpox infection anywhere in the world for the past twenty-five years.

Federal grant money, under President Bush's multimillion-dollar Project BioShield program, has been allocated to technologic innovation for bioterrorism prevention. By 2003, according to The Chronicle of Higher Education, the National Institutes of Health were supporting almost seventy extramural research projects on anthrax alone. The NIH has funded two new National Biocontainment Laboratories and new facilities at Regional Biocontainment Laboratories, most at major universities, to the tune of $360 million in start-up costs. The University of Pittsburgh just lured the top staff of the Center for Civilian Biodefense Strategies away from Johns Hopkins by offering to set up a Center for Biosecurity with a

$12 million endowment. The University of South Florida recently received $5 million in federal grant money for its Center for Biological Defense, which has projects like "Photocatalytic Air Disinfection" and "Aquatic Real-time Monitoring System (ARMS) for Bioterrorism Events." And Auburn University received a million-dollar federal biopreparedness grant for something called a Canine Detection Center.

When Harvard received a $1.2 million federal grant in 2002 to set up a program for detecting "events possibly related to bioterrorism" by electronically linking 20 million patient-care records from around the country (an endeavor called syndromic surveillance), the grant was a mere drop in the bucket: Congress soon allotted $420 million to Homeland Security for a larger linked health-monitoring network. A consortium led by the New York Academy of Medicine then developed software for syndromic surveillance. The new software allows public health officials to monitor what are called "aberrant clusters health events"—translation: more than the expected number of cases of some symptom that might be related to a disease that might be produced by an organism that might be in the possession of terrorists. Syndromic surveillance works fine if someone knows what to look for. But it is of no help at all with the unexpected. When there really was bioterrorism in the U.S.—the anthrax attacks in fall 2001—linked databases were useless; it took a smart clinician to figure out that anthrax was around, and old-fashioned shoe-leather epidemiology quickly worked out which people had been affected. West Nile virus, ditto. A friend who is an official of a local health department tells me that the syndromic surveillance experts find it works well for predicting the first influenza outbreak each year. But anyone's grandmother can predict the first influenza outbreak where I live, in the New York City area, since the symptoms are always the same and flu always starts here in the two weeks preceding Thanksgiving. For all its meager productivity, the syndromic surveillance software also throws out plenty of false-positive "clusters" that waste investigator's time. It is our new and expensive white elephant, justified by the fear of evildoers and germs.

It all sounds a little phantasmagoric.

In The Exposé of 1935, Walter Benjamin identified certain phantasmagorias of modern life as Wunschbilder, "wish symbols," that seek to "transfigure the . . . inadequacies in the social organization." Benjamin was concerned with phantasmagorias as magical images, as he put it in his Passagen-Werk, "residues of a dream world," revelations of unfulfilled wishes. In this sense we might ask whether the many projects of the Bioshield—the electronic anthrax detectors, the hyperdatabanks, the supersecure biohazard-level-4 labs, the men and women in full-body protective suits, the urban-evacuation exercises, whatever it is they are doing with dogs at Auburn University, and so on—are emblems of some shared desire to feel that all the effort America expends on technology development protects us from something. We might ask whether the something is the Stranger Spreading Germs. And we must ask what the cost is.

The core issue here is that the Stranger Spreading Germs is a metaphor, and largely an empty one. Bioterrorism is not a public-health problem, and will not become one. The next plague, whatever it is, will not decimate us unheralded. In signing the contract on biopreparedness, we have bought a confection, a defense against the chimeric stranger with the metaphorical germs.

And the costs of buy-in? When our public-health "leaders" corroborate government rhetoric about bioterrorists by reassuring us that our state or municipal health department is ready for any smallpox, anthrax, or plague attack, they legitimate both their own efforts and the standing of their offices. The planned result is that we will not question spending tax dollars so those officials can continue to defend us, even when it means closing down municipal clinics or shortchanging programs for the poor, and even if such biodefense is not what we most need or want.

The biopreparedness campaign goes to work. It discredits the simple logic of public health. Lose the distinction between the minuscule risk of dying in an intentional outbreak and the millionfold-higher chance of dying in a natural pandemic, it says. Ignore the hundredfold-higher-still chance of dying of cancer or heart disease. Defund the prenatal-care clinics, the chest clinics, the exercise and cancer screening and lead abatement programs. Ignore the lessons of history: forget that human attempts to create epidemics have almost always failed, and dismiss the repeated ability of a well-funded public-health apparatus to control epidemic disease with time-tested measures. Just think about germs, and tremble.

The lesson of history that we ignore at our peril is this: nobody can tell us how the next epidemic will happen. New germs come and go, epidemics wax and wane, but national catastrophes happen rarely. And when they do, it is never because of a stranger spreading germs. Anyone who promises certain protection from the next plague is selling us a bill of goods.

Biological Weapons

FOREIGN POLICY, SEPTEMBER/OCTOBER 2006

After 9/11, U.S. spending on defenses against biological attacks got a shot in the arm. Between 2001 and 2006, the budget for biodefense medical research and development at the National Institutes of Health increased from $50 million to $1.8 billion. Five years later, it turns out there might be some unlikely beneficiaries of this bounty: poor people in the developing world.

The extra money being poured into bioterror preparedness could result in a revolution in global public health—to the benefit of the world's most vulnerable citizens. New vaccines, medicines, and techniques designed to deal with diseases unleashed by terrorists may also combat naturally occurring outbreaks. Tara O'Toole, director of the Center for Biosecurity at the University of Pittsburgh Medical Center and a former assistant secretary of energy, argues that "if we do what is necessary for biodefense . . . we could conceivably in a generation eliminate large-scale, lethal epidemics of infectious disease everywhere."

Vaccines are notoriously unprofitable, so pharmaceutical companies have often shown little interest in developing them. But fears of a biological attack have led the U.S. government to fund new vaccine breakthroughs for ebola, the Marburg virus, and Lassa fever. This money will also speed the development of dengue fever and vibrio cholera vaccines. Scientists are also excited about the possibilities stemming from the military's bigger budgets. Steven Block, a Stanford University scientist who has consulted for the U.S. government on national security, says that "the military has, literally, billions of dollars burning a hole in its pocket for spending on things biomedical." He's confident that any benefits will be shared with the public at large: "This doesn't strike me as the kind of thing that the military would develop and then keep top secret."

Still, O'Toole frets that the research might be conducted as "fortress America, with a very narrow focus on countering weapons," limiting the public-health benefits. Also, it costs more than a billion dollars to bring a new vaccine to market. That means that the level of success "comes down to how wisely they do or don't spend this money," says Block. Ironically, sharing these medical advances with the world could help win the war they were designed to fight in the first place.

Pox Unlocked?

By Ingrid Wickelgren
Current Science, March 18, 2005

Should scientists be allowed to tinker with the smallpox virus?

When medical researchers go to work at a lab in Atlanta, they don blue hazmat suits to protect themselves against their subject: the Variola virus. Variola is the highly contagious germ that causes smallpox, one of history's worst mass murderers.

Today, nobody gets smallpox, thanks to a World Health Organization (WHO) campaign that wiped out the disease in the 1970s. But scientists in two laboratories—one at the Centers for Disease Control and Prevention (CDC) in Atlanta and the other in Russia—still experiment with the Variola virus. Last fall, a WHO committee recommended that the scientists also be permitted to genetically engineer the virus to create a mutant form of it. Genetic engineering is the manipulation of an organism's genes.

Many scientists think such tinkering is too dangerous. Others say it is necessary to protect the world from potential outbreaks of the disease.

Pro

Scientists who support the WHO proposal say it could speed the development of treatments in the event of a terrorist attack involving smallpox. Some U.S. government officials are concerned that terrorists may have illegally obtained the smallpox virus from a Russian lab. The Russian government once made biological weapons—weapons devised to infect people or animals with harmful germs.

At the CDC, researchers are trying to develop smallpox antivirals (drugs that treat diseases caused by viruses) as well as faster ways of diagnosing smallpox. The researchers are also trying to develop better animal models for the testing of treatments and new vaccines, says Inger Damon, chief of the CDC Poxvirus Section. Animal models are animals that can develop a disease that is similar to a disease that afflicts humans. Treatments meant for people can first be tried on the animal models.

Damon says some genetic alterations of the smallpox virus will speed that research. One CDC proposal calls for inserting a green fluorescent protein into the virus so that living viruses will glow.

Any virus killed by a drug would no longer glow green, making it easy to tell if the drug works against the virus. This tactic, says Damon, would result in "more efficient screening [testing] of antivirals" and quicken the development of smallpox treatments.

Security is extremely tight around the smallpox lab at the CDC. Since 1980, the smallpox virus has been held in a maximum-containment biosafety level 4 lab, otherwise known as a "suit lab." "The danger of working with the virus is that it will escape," Thomas Mack, a smallpox expert at the University of Southern California, told Current Science. "That's not going to happen at the CDC."

"The virus can be used for bioterrorism," said Llelwyn Grant, a CDC spokesperson. "Because of that, we feel that it is important to continue with research so that the American public is protected."

Con

Many researchers oppose the WHO proposal. They believe that tinkering with the genome (genetic material) of the smallpox virus poses unacceptable risks.

Case in point: To insert the green protein, scientists must first find a stable point in the virus's genome. If the point's location were to be publicized in a scientific journal, an unscrupulous scientist who illegally possesses the smallpox virus could use the information to insert a dangerous gene into the virus, says Jens Kuhn, a virologist at Harvard Medical School in Boston. The result might be, say, an, even more contagious form of smallpox.

Why not keep the location secret? That would only anger other scientists, says Kuhn. All research results are normally shared with other scientists so they can build on the work. Officials from other countries might worry if the United States kept secrets about smallpox. "No matter what they do, there will be problems," said Kuhn.

The WHO has also proposed that smallpox researchers be allowed to insert Variola virus genes into other similar types of viruses. But, opponents say, that might result in a deadly new virus. "You do not know what you will get," Kuhn warned. "From a security standpoint, I am concerned about it."

Opponents also say that the benefits of manipulating the smallpox virus's genes aren't worth the risks. After all, nobody is suffering from smallpox now, and no one may ever again. "The fear [of smallpox] is in our minds," said biologist Sujatha Byravan, executive director of the Council for Responsible Genetics, in Cambridge, Mass. "The risks of experimentation are not justified by the need."

Donald Henderson, the doctor and scientist who led the WHO smallpox eradication campaign in the 1970s, also questions the practicality of developing smallpox treatments. The price tag will be at least $800 million, he says. Who is going to pay for that? "That's the question to answer," Henderson opined.

Henderson and others say the WHO should demand that Russia and the United States destroy the smallpox virus by a certain date. Refusal to do so would be considered a crime against humanity, he says. "This would lessen the likelihood that people would have the virus," Henderson argued.

Identifying Airborne Pathogens in Time to Respond

BY GABRIELE RENNIE
SCIENCE & TECHNOLOGY REVIEW, OCTOBER 2005

Among the possible terrorist activities that might threaten national security is the release of an airborne pathogen such as anthrax. Because the potential damage to human health could be severe, experts consider 1 minute to be an operationally useful time limit for identifying the pathogen and taking action. Many commercial systems can identify airborne pathogenic microbes, but they take days or, at best, hours to produce results. The Department of Homeland Security (DHS) and other U.S. government agencies are interested in finding a faster approach.

To answer this national need, a Livermore team, led by scientist Eric Gard, has developed the bioaerosol mass spectrometry (BAMS) system—the only instrument that can detect and identify spores at low concentrations in less than 1 minute BAMS can successfully distinguish between two related but different spore species. It can also sort out a single spore from thousands of other particles—biological and nonbioiogical—with no false positives (See *S&TR*, September 2003, pp. 21–23.)

The BAMS team won a 2005 R&D 100 Award for developing the system. Livermore's Laboratory Directed Research and Development (LDRD) Program funded the biomedical aspects of the BAMS project, and the Department of Defense's Technical Support Working Group and Defense Advanced Research Project Agency funded the biodefense efforts.

Developing a detection system that can analyze small samples so quickly has been challenging. Livermore engineer Vincent Riot, who worked on the BAMS project, explains, "A typical spore weighs approximately one-trillionth of a gram and is dispersed in the atmosphere, which contains naturally occurring particles that could be present at concentrations thousands of times higher. Previous systems also had difficulty separating benign organisms from those that are pathogenic but very similar, which has resulted in false alarms."

Credit is given to the University of California, Lawrence Livermore National Laboratory, and the Department of Energy under whose auspices the work was performed.

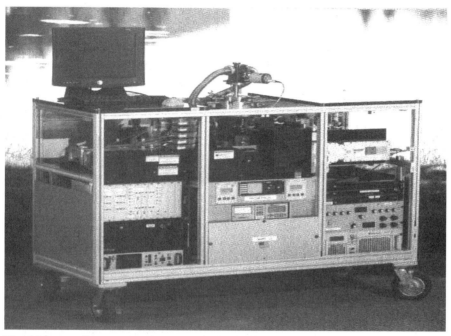

The bioaerosol mass spectrometry (BAMS) system—about the size of three lecterns—can identify bioagents, such as anthrax, and it has the potential to differentiate between normal and cancerous cells.

Sorting Between Harmful and Benign

BAMS operates by drawing air through a nozzle and removing nearly all the particles too small to be biological threat agents. The remaining particles—each about 0.5 to 10 micrometers in diameter—are focused into a tight beam. A particle accelerates to a velocity determined by its size and shape, which provides information on a particle's type. The system then probes each particle to determine if it contains biological material. For this operation, a pulsed-laser beam excites the particles. Biological materials, if present, emit fluorescent light, which can be recorded by the detector, but nonbiological particles, such as dirt in the atmosphere, do not emit light. This step reduces the number of particles for further analysis by 90 percent.

In the system's final step, a mass spectrometer identifies the particles. Most mass spectrometers operate by measuring either positive or negative ions. BAMS uses a dual-polarity mass spectrometer, which can process a particle's positive and negative ions at the same time. The positive and negative ions formed are further separated by polarity and mass-to-charge ratio. Real-time pattern-recognition software developed at the Laboratory then analyzes and categorizes the resulting spectra. Every organism produces a unique signature, which BAMS compares with spectra in a database of organisms.

The system can analyze thousands of particles per second, so it can distinguish a very small concentration of biological aerosol from a much larger concentration of background aerosol.

To test the system, the Livermore team used *Bacillus subtilis var. niger*, a surrogate of anthrax (*B. anthracis*), and *B. thuringiensis*, an organic pesticide that differs from *B. anthracis* in two short sections of its DNA. BAMS successfully distinguished between the two. The instrument also identified other bacterial cells and spores, biological toxins, and viruses. "BAMS is the only system that can identity harmful biological agents in enough time to evacuate an area," says Riot, "and it can do so with almost no false positives, which is essential in reducing the panic that alarms can cause."

In a recent study, the team placed BAMS in the international terminal at San Francisco International Airport to help DHS determine the cause for false positives registered by other equipment. The instrument has also been used in preliminary studies at Livermore's Site 300, where BAMS successfully distinguished particles in the atmosphere and surrounding soil from those generated by a detonation of conventional high explosives.

The system's ability to analyze particles or cells could benefit other fields in addition to biological threat detection. Potential applications include medical diagnostics, explosives detection, meteorological studies, and nonproliferation programs. For example, the BAMS team hopes to build on the Site 300 research to develop detection capabilities for radioisotopes, which would benefit the nation's nonproliferation programs.

Detecting Communicable Airborne Diseases

BAMS also has the potential to detect communicable diseases such as severe acute respiratory syndrome (SARS) or tuberculosis, which typically take about a week for clinical detection. Livermore researchers have used tuberculosis surrogates to test the system's ability in this area. The LDRD Program is funding an effort to analyze human sputum. Led by physicist Matthias Frank, the project includes researchers from the Laboratory's Chemistry and Materials Science; Physics and Advanced Technologies; Nonproliferation, Arms Control, and International Security; and Biosciences directorates. By learning which particles occur naturally, these scientists hope to find a method for detecting abnormal cells for various diseases. Riot says, "The idea is to have a person breathe into a mask, then let BAMS analyze the particles released from the lungs and identify them instantaneously."

The current BAMS system, about the size of three lecterns, is available for licensing. The Livermore team continues to work on improving the system's capability and reducing its size to fit various needs. Whether used to detect biological agents or contagious diseases, BAMS shows great promise for identifying problems reliably when time is of the essence.

Bid to Stockpile Bioterror Drugs Stymied by Setbacks

By Eric Lipton
THE NEW YORK TIMES, SEPTEMBER 18, 2006

The last of the anthrax-laced letters was still making its way through the mail in late 2001 when top Bush administration officials reached an obvious conclusion: the nation desperately needed to expand its medical stockpile to prepare for another biological attack.

The result was Project BioShield, a $5.6 billion effort to exploit the country's top medical and scientific brains and fill an emergency medical cabinet with new drugs and vaccines for a host of threats. "We will rally the great promise of American science and innovation to confront the greatest danger of our time," President Bush said in starting the program.

But the project, critics say, has largely failed to deliver.

So far, only a small fraction of the anticipated remedies are available. Drug companies have waited months, if not years, for government agencies to decide which treatments they want and in what quantities. Unable to attract large pharmaceutical corporations to join the endeavor, the government is instead relying on small start-up companies that often have no proven track record.

The troubles have been most acute with the highest priority of all: a $900 million push to add a new anthrax vaccine to the stockpile. What had begun as an effort to test and manufacture a safer, faster-acting vaccine has turned into an ugly battle between two biotech businesses.

Each has hired Washington lobbyists to attack its rival's product and try to win over lawmakers and administration officials. Delivery of the new vaccine is far behind schedule, and a dispute between the Department of Health and Human Services and VaxGen, the company chosen to make the vaccine, could even end the deal. The only doses that have been added to the stockpile are of a decades-old vaccine that has generated complaints of serious side effects.

Health department officials acknowledge some problems but say they have made progress. "Medical discovery is an unpredictable process," said Bill Hall, a spokesman. "It is the nature of science."

But some companies on the sidelines say the experience with the anthrax vaccine is exactly why they do not want to do business with Washington. Once optimistic about the president's promise, many biotech companies and public health experts are now discouraged.

"The inept implementation of the program has led the best brains and the best scientists to give up, to look elsewhere or devote their resources to medical initiatives that are not focused on biodefense," said Michael Greenberger, director of the Center for Health and Homeland Security at the University of Maryland.

Even some former department officials who helped create Bio-Shield are dismayed.

"I find this all rather repugnant," said D. A. Henderson, a former top bioterrorism official. "You have people here who, in the face of a problem of serious import, are using every tactic they can to line their own pockets."

Risk and Disappointment

From the start, officials in Washington knew that Project Bio-Shield would be a risky venture—for the government, the companies involved and even ordinary Americans, who might be asked to take relatively untested treatments in an emergency.

Officials hoped $5.6 billion in federal money would entice companies to develop new drugs and vaccines for anthrax, smallpox, botulism, Ebola and other deadly diseases.

Because of the perceived urgency of the threat, the project suspends some traditional standards. It allows new vaccines or drugs to be used in emergencies before completing the lengthy Food and Drug Administration approval process. Full testing on humans is also not required because it is too dangerous, even though that means no one will know with certainty whether the vaccines will work until used in a crisis.

For their part, the companies have to take all the risks of developing and manufacturing new products; they get paid only upon delivery.

At the top of the government's threat list was anthrax, which killed five people, created panic and disrupted the mail system after letters filled with the powder were sent through the mail. No one has been charged in the attacks, which affected places including a tabloid publication in Florida, a New York television network and several lawmakers' offices on Capitol Hill.

"The top three threats, in fact, are anthrax, anthrax, anthrax," Dr. Gerald Parker, a senior health agency official, said in an interview. If properly dispersed through the air, just a few hundred pounds of anthrax powder could endanger tens of thousands of people.

After the letter attacks, the health agency bought enough antibiotics for 41 million Americans, but the recommended treatment augments those drugs with a vaccine. The government already had an anthrax vaccine to inoculate military personnel, but it involved six shots over 18 months, an unusually long course of treatment. While the F.D.A. says it is safe and effective, it can have nasty side effects. There have been reports among military personnel of six deaths and serious complications, including lymphoma and multiple sclerosis. The military stopped mandatory vaccinations in 2004 after some soldiers balked and filed lawsuits.

"It is 1950's technology," said Dr. Philip K. Russell, the former acting director of the office that started Project BioShield. "We don't drive Model T Fords anymore."

The first disappointment with the new anthrax vaccine occurred in early 2004 when bids to test and manufacture it came in. None were from big pharmaceutical companies; they considered the effort unappealing because the potential market was relatively small and profits limited. They were also concerned about liability if someone became ill or died after being inoculated. Project BioShield did not offer immunity from lawsuits.

That left a handful of companies in the running, relatively small outfits with limited experience. VaxGen, for example, had never taken a drug to market. Its first major product, an AIDS vaccine, flopped in 2003. The company also had financial troubles; it was barred from Nasdaq in 2004 after managers uncovered accounting errors.

The situation was hardly ideal, federal health officials acknowledged.

"We are going to be working consistently with these smaller firms, and it's going to require an enormous amount of government effort to get this product licensed," said Stewart Simonson, then an assistant health secretary overseeing the anthrax vaccine effort.

VaxGen argues that a company does not have to be large to successfully produce a vaccine. "We've repeatedly demonstrated that we have the capacity, expertise and infrastructure to meet the government's needs," said Lance Ignon, a vice president of the company, which is based in Brisbane, Calif.

Instead of hedging its bets by dividing the work among several vendors, Health and Human Services awarded the entire $887 million order to VaxGen. It was to produce 75 million doses, enough to inoculate 25 million Americans.

That decision fed doubts about Project BioShield in Congress and drew loud complaints that would grow into sharp opposition from Emergent BioSolutions, the maker of the old vaccine, which is based in Gaithersburg, Md.

Then known as BioPort and based in Lansing, Mich., the company did not submit a bid for the new vaccine. Instead, it had been trying for months to persuade the federal government to buy hundreds of millions of dollars of the existing vaccine, its only major product. When executives learned that one competitor was getting all the work, they knew the company's future was in peril.

[VaxGen] had never taken a drug to market. Its first major product, an AIDS vaccine, flopped in 2003.

Soon, though, they found an important weapon for a campaign to recapture business.

Competition Heats Up

VaxGen's vaccine was based on a modified version of the old one; Army scientists had genetically re-engineered it in hopes of making it safer and faster, with three shots instead of six. But VaxGen tests in early 2005 showed that an ingredient added to the vaccine caused it to decompose. It would not survive long in the emergency stockpile.

VaxGen officials played down the setback, which delayed delivery to 2007 from 2006. "We are being called on to develop a vaccine in roughly half the time it normally takes," Mr. Ignon said. "When you do that, you have to accept the fact that there are going to be some unexpected turns."

But Emergent officials capitalized on VaxGen's stumble. They had already gotten health agency officials to agree to buy five million doses of their vaccine to add to the stockpile. Now they began pushing for a much larger deal, possibly replacing VaxGen's vaccine altogether, company documents show.

To lead its lobbying effort, which has cost more than $1 million since 2005, Emergent turned to Jerome M. Hauer, a top official at the health department until late 2003. While at the agency, he supported the push for a new vaccine. Now he was trying to persuade Congress and his former employer to buy the old vaccine.

Explaining his shift, Mr. Hauer said VaxGen's problems convinced him that Emergent's vaccine was the best choice. In retrospect, he said, "The advice we were given was wrong."

Emergent hired nearly a dozen other lobbyists, some of whom had similarly useful connections. They included John M. Clerici, a lawyer who had helped shape the BioShield legislation; John Hishta, former chief of staff to Representative Thomas M. Davis III, Republican of Virginia; and Allen Shofe, a former tobacco industry lobbyist.

The lobbyists argued that quality control problems at Emergent's plant in Michigan had been corrected and that reports of serious side effects from the vaccine were unfounded. But mostly, they tried to undermine confidence in VaxGen.

In a series of meetings with lawmakers and administration officials, they attacked their rival. "VaxGen has a history of failure and irregularities," their briefing books said. "VaxGen has never produced an F.D.A.–approved product," and its "vaccine is based on unproven technology," leaving "the health and protection of the American public on a company with a history of scientific failure and financial scandal."

The lobbyists also criticized the officials involved in administering BioShield. In speeches and news interviews, Mr. Hauer questioned the credentials of Mr. Simonson, the health department official in charge of the program, and once called him the "Mike Brown of

H.H.S.," a reference to the disgraced former director of the Federal Emergency Management Agency. (Mr. Simonson, who resigned this year, had worked as an Amtrak lawyer and as legal counsel to Gov. Tommy G. Thompson of Wisconsin, who was later head of the federal health department.)

> Threatening to sue, VaxGen is seeking upfront payments from the health department or other concessions.

The lobbyists also charged that Dr. Russell, who helped start Project BioShield, had a conflict of interest. They said he had helped develop the vaccine as former director of the Walter Reed Army Institute of Research and then been instrumental in awarding the manufacturing contract after moving to the health department. (Dr. Russell says he retired from the Army before it began research on the Vax-Gen vaccine.)

Fearful of losing the public relations battle, VaxGen increased its own lobbying effort. It hired Robert Housman, who had worked with Mr. Hauer to help Emergent open its anti-VaxGen campaign and then switched sides. But VaxGen, which spent $200,000 on lobbying last year, was outmanned by Emergent and put on the defensive.

Senator Charles E. Grassley, an Iowa Republican and focus of Emergent's lobbying, sent a letter to Health and Human Services Secretary Michael O. Leavitt that closely echoed criticisms of Vax-Gen that had first been raised in Emergent documents.

Representative Davis scheduled a hearing last summer at which Emergent's chief executive was invited to testify, but no one was invited from VaxGen. Mr. Davis said Mr. Hishta, his former aide, apparently did contact his office about Emergent. But he said he was not sure why only Emergent was asked to testify.

Under pressure from Congress, the health agency agreed in May to double its order of Emergent's vaccine to 10 million doses, worth $243 million. The next day, health officials demanded what VaxGen says are additional safety and efficacy tests that will further delay delivery by a year or two. Threatening to sue, VaxGen is seeking upfront payments from the health department or other concessions. If no agreement is reached, company officials say, the entire deal could collapse.

"We understand this program is new and changes will have to be made," said Piers Whitehead, a vice president of VaxGen. "But in our case, the goalposts were moved much farther than they needed to be."

Words of Determination

Health officials said they were determined to see the anthrax contract—and other BioShield endeavors—through to the end.

"There are people out there who feel like they are not getting a piece of the pie or that this is not running the right way," said Mr. Hall, the department spokesman. "That may be. But to come in and criticize BioShield as a failing program because we have not spent all the money and don't have all the products in the warehouse is completely and sorely misguided."

The maneuvering has been so intense, with lobbyists and media consultants helping the companies undermine the competition, even some of the people who have profited now express disgust.

"This ought be driven by the science, by efficacy and threat, not lobbyists," Mr. Housman said. "It has been shanghaied. And the implication is our national security is compromised."

Next week, agency officials will meet with industry representatives to discuss a new strategy for Project BioShield. Mr. Greenberger, the University of Maryland expert, and others argue that government agencies must determine more quickly what is needed for the stockpile and provide more financial incentives to lure the big companies and better support the start-up companies.

Some in Congress say the improvements are much needed because Project BioShield has proven so disappointing.

"A torturous labyrinth of federal fiefdoms into which billions disappear," Representative Christopher Shays, Republican of Connecticut, said of the program. "Yet few antidotes have yet to emerge."

The Biodefense Buildup

Fallout for Other Research Areas?

By Barton Reppert
Bioscience, April 2005

Massive expansion of the US biodefense program since 2001 has yielded fresh career opportunities for thousands of American scientists handling infectious disease work. With the Bush administration determined to develop better countermeasures against bioterrorism, this trend is likely to continue for the next several years.

However, the rapid buildup of new laboratories, personnel, and funding for biodefense could have a significant downside for other important areas of research—and, some scientists contend, may actually contribute to the erosion of this country's public health infrastructure.

The fiscal year (FY) 2006 federal budget, sent to Congress on 7 February, signaled President George W. Bush's intention to keep pouring money into biodefense. "We have spent or requested nearly $19.2 billion since September 11, 2001," Secretary of Health and Human Services Mike Leavitt told reporters, "and that investment is showing tangible results."

According to research analyst Ari Schuler at the University of Pittsburgh Center for Biosecurity, in the current fiscal year, combined spending for civilian biodefense by seven federal departments and agencies is estimated to total about $7.647 billion—approximately 18 times more than FY 2001 outlays of $414 million.

One of the results of the steeply ramped-up biodefense effort is a network of new, high-security laboratories for research on infectious diseases. The network, funded by the National Institute of Allergy and Infectious Diseases (NIAID), a part of the National Institutes of Health (NIH), will comprise two large national biocontainment laboratories (to be built at Boston University's Medical Center and at the University of Texas Medical Branch in Galveston), along with 14 to 17 smaller regional biocontainment laboratories. The two national facilities will include a substantial amount of biosafety level 4 (BSL-4) laboratory space, while the regional facilities will feature BSL-3 and BSL-2 labs. In addition, NIAID is funding the establishment of 10 Regional Centers of Excellence for Biodefense and Emerging Infectious Diseases Research, each of which comprises a consortium of universities and complementary research institutions, to support the NIAID biodefense research agenda.

Proponents of that agenda, including Dr. Anthony Fauci, director of NIAID, argue that biodefense research represents money well spent because it is dual-purpose: it is valuable not only for developing better vaccines, diagnostics, and therapeutics against bioterrorist agents but also for coping with naturally occurring infectious diseases. Several critics within the scientific community, however, contend that the biodefense effort is largely a politically motivated overreaction—following the fall 2001 anthrax-by-mail incidents—to a limited threat.

One outspoken critic, Richard Ebright, a molecular biologist and professor of chemistry and chemical biology at Rutgers University, has initiated and circulated to colleagues an open letter to Elias Zerhouni, NIH director, charging that the priority placed on biodefense

---

"The threat of a mass-casualty bioterrorist attack has been greatly overestimated."—Mark Wheelis, biological weapons expert, University of California, Davis

---

research since 2001 has been accompanied by "a massive efflux of funding, institutions, and investigators from work on non-biodefense-related microbial physiology, genetics, and pathogenesis."

The letter, signed by more than 750 researchers, says the number of grants awarded by NIAID referencing "prioritized bioweapons agents" has increased by 1500 percent, from 33 in 1996–2000 to 497 since 2001. By contrast, grants awarded to study non-biodefense-related model microorganisms have decreased by 41 percent over the same period, from 490 down to 289, while grants to study non-biodefense-related pathogenic microorganisms have decreased by 27 percent, from 627 down to 457.

"The diversion of research funds from projects of high public-health importance to projects of high biodefense but low public-health importance represents a misdirection of NIH priorities and a crisis for NIH-supported microbiological research," declares the scientists' letter, urging that Zerhouni "take corrective action."

Another critic of the biodefense buildup, Mark Wheelis, an expert on biological weapons at the University of California at Davis, says he believes that "the threat of a mass-casualty bioterrorist attack has been greatly overestimated. The possibility of such an attack is clearly not zero, but it's probably quite a bit less likely than many people think." Regarding the new network of biocontainment laboratories, Wheelis observes that "a small increase in our capacity to do work on very serious pathogens under high containment is reasonable. . . . But plastering the country with BSL-3 and BSL-4 labs is going to degrade our public health infrastructure more than it will aid it."

The Bush administration has renewed its resolve to move ahead with a heavily funded fight against the perceived threat of bioterrorism. At the same time, it is clear that the continuing biodefense buildup will not only involve "hot zone" pathogens but also generate a substantial amount of heated debate within the American scientific community.

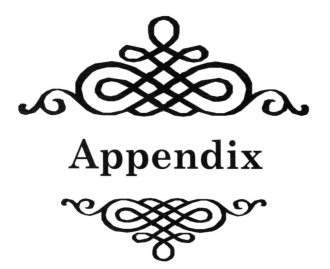

Appendix

25 Years of AIDS

UN Chronicle, June/August 2006

In June 1981, scientists in the United States reported the first clinical evidence of a disease that would later become known as acquired immunodeficiency syndrome or AIDS. Twenty-five years later, the AIDS epidemic has spread to every corner of the world. Around 40 million people today are living with HIV and over 25 million have died of the disease. But years of struggle to control the epidemic have also yielded a growing list of breakthroughs.

1959

- The oldest specimen of the human immunodeficiency virus (HIV) ever detected in a blood sample—donated by a man in Leopoldville, Congo.

1981

- The first cases of unusual immune system failures are identified among gay men, women and injecting drug users.

1982

- AIDS is defined for the first time. In the course of the year, the three modes of transmission are identified: blood, mother-to-child and sexual intercourse.

1983

- Dr. Luc Montagnier in France isolates lymphadenopathy-associated virus (LAV), later to become known as human immunodeficiency virus or HIV.
- A heterosexual AIDS epidemic is revealed in Central Africa.

1984

- Dr. Robert Gallo in the United States identifies HIV as the cause of AIDS.

1985

- The global scope of the growing epidemic becomes manifest. By 1985, at least one case of HIV has been reported in each region of the world.

- The first HIV antibody tests are commercialized in the United States and in Europe, and HIV screening of blood donations begins.

- More than 2,000 people attend the first international conference on AIDS in Atlanta.

- A clinical case definition of AIDS is developed for developing countries at a World Health Organization (WHO) workshop on AIDS in Bangui, Central African Republic.

- American film star Rock Hudson becomes the first international icon to disclose he has AIDS.

1986

- The International Steering Committee for People with HIV/AIDS is created—later to become the Global Network of People Living with HIV/AIDS (GNP+).

1987

- Africa's first community-based response to AIDS (The AIDS Support Organisation or TASO) is formed in Uganda. It becomes a role model for similar groups around the world.

- In February, WHO establishes the Special Programme on AIDS.

- AIDS becomes the first disease ever debated on the floor of the United Nations General Assembly.

- The first therapy for AIDS—azidothymidine (AZT)—is approved for use in the United States.

1988

- The International AIDS Society is founded—an organization of professionals working on HIV/AIDS.

- Health ministers from around the world meet in London and discuss the AIDS epidemic for the first time.

- WHO declares 1 December as World AIDS Day.

- Women account for half of adults living with HIV in sub-Saharan Africa (as assessed by recent models through national surveys).

1990

- By 1990 around 1 million children have lost one or both parents to AIDS.

1991

- The red ribbon becomes an international symbol of AIDS awareness.

- The global network of non-governmental and community-based organizations—International Council of AIDS Service Organization (ICASO)—is formed to mobilize communities and their organizations to participate in the response to AIDS.

1992–1993

- HIV prevalence in Uganda and Thailand begins to decrease as a result of countrywide mobilization against the epidemic.

1994

- At the Paris AIDS Summit, 42 national governments declare that the principle of greater involvement of people living with HIV (GIPA) is critical to ethical and effective national responses to the epidemic.
- Scientists develop the first treatment regimen to reduce mother-to-child HIV transmission.

1995

- An HIV outbreak in Eastern Europe is detected among injecting drug users.

1996

- The Joint United Nations Programme on HIV/AIDS (UNAIDS) becomes operational.
- Evidence of the efficacy of highly active antiretroviral (ART) therapy presented for the first time at the 11th International AIDS Conference in Vancouver.
- Brazil becomes the first developing country to provide ART through its public health system.

1997

- With the support of UNAIDS, the first public ART programme in Africa, the Drug Access Initiative, is launched first in Kampala and later in Abidjan.
- The Global Business Council on HIV/AIDS is created (later to become the Global Business Coalition on AIDS).
- USAID publishes the first "Children on the Brink: Strategies to Support HIV/AIDS" report, highlighting the epidemic's impact on children.

1998

- The first short-course regimen to prevent mother-to-child transmission is announced.
- The Treatment Action Campaign (TAC) is established in South Africa to mobilize national support for people living with HIV to access treatments.

- Thirty-nine pharmaceutical companies file a law suit against the South African Government to contest legislation aimed at reducing the price of medicines.

1999

- The first efficacy trial of a potential HIV vaccine in a developing country starts in Thailand.
- The UN launches the International Partnership against AIDS in Africa, to bring together key stakeholders to mount an intensified response to the epidemic.

2000

- The UN Security Council discusses AIDS for the first time.
- The Millennium Development Goals, which include reversing the spread of AIDS, tuberculosis and malaria among the eight key targets, are announced as part of the Millennium Declaration.
- UNAIDS and WHO announce a joint initiative—the Accelerating Access Initiative—with five pharmaceutical companies to increase access to HIV treatment in developing countries.

2001

- Secretary-General Kofi Annan launches a call to action in Abuja, requesting for a "war chest" of $7 million to $10 billion to be spent annually on AIDS in developing countries.
- The first General Assembly Special Session on HIV/AIDS unanimously adopts the Declaration of Commitment on HIV/AIDS, which declares AIDS a global catastrophe and calls for worldwide commitment to fight the disease.
- The World Trade Organization adopts the Doha Declaration, allowing for wider access to HIV treatment through generic drugs.

2002

- The Global Fund to Fight AIDS, Tuberculosis and Malaria becomes operational and approves the first round of grants.

2003

- United States President George Bush announces the $15-billion President's Emergency Plan for AIDS Relief during the State of the Union address.
- WHO and UNAIDS launch the "3 by 5" initiative with the aim of helping low- and middle-income countries increase the number of people who have access to antiretroviral therapy from 400,000 to 3 million people by the end of 2005.

2004

- UNAIDS launches the Global Coalition on Women and AIDS.

- An agreement is reached on the "Three Ones" principle—one national AIDS framework, one national AIDS authority and one system for monitoring and evaluation—as the guiding principles for engagement on AIDS by national and international actors.

2005

- At the G-8 Summit in Gleneagles, Scotland, leaders pledge to come as close as possible to universal access to ART worldwide by 2010.

- At the United Nations 2005 World Summit in New York, world leaders agree to take action to scale up HIV prevention, treatment, care and support, with the aim of coming as close as possible to the goal of universal access to treatment by 2010 for all those who need it.

- Indian Prime Minister Manmohan Singh establishes the National Council on AIDS.

- Chinese Premier Wen Jiabao announces increased measures to fight AIDS.

- A "Global Task Team on improving coordination among multilateral institutions and international donors to further strengthen the AIDS response in countries" recommends measures to improve effectiveness of the international response to AIDS.

- UNICEF and UNAIDS launch "Unite for Children, Unite Against AIDS—a global campaign focusing on the enormous impact of AIDS on children.

- By the end of 2005, 1.3 million people in low-and middle-income countries are receiving access to antiretroviral therapy.

Source: UNAIDS, *2006 Report on the global AIDS epidemic*

Bibliography

Books

Barnard, Bryn. *Outbreak: Plagues that Changed History*. New York: Crown Publishers, 2005.

Barry, John M. *The Great Influenza: The Epic Story of the Greatest Plague in History*. New York: Viking Penguin, 2004.

Benedictow, Ole J. *The Black Death, 1346–1353: The Complete History*. Rochester, N.Y.: Boydell Press, 2004.

Crosby, Alfred W. *America's Forgotten Pandemic: The Influenza of 1918*. Cambridge: Cambridge University Press, 1990.

Crosby, Molly Caldwell. *The American Plague: The Untold Story of Yellow Fever, the Epidemic that Shaped Our History*. New York: Berkley Books, 2006.

DeSalle, Rob, ed. *Epidemic!: The World of Infectious Diseases*. New York: The New Press, 1999.

Diamond, Jared M. *Guns, Germs, and Steel*. New York: W. W. Norton & Co., 1997.

Dormandy, Thomas. *The White Death: A History of Tuberculosis*. Rio Grande, Ohio: Hambledon Press, 1999.

Drexler, Madeline. *Secret Agents: The Menace of Emerging Infections*. Washington, D.C.: Joseph Henry Press, 2002.

Engel, Jonathan. *The Epidemic: A Global History of AIDS*. New York: Smithsonian Books/Collins, 2006.

Garrett, Laurie. *The Coming Plague: Newly Emerging Diseases in a World out of Balance*. New York: Farrar, Straus and Giroux, 1994.

Hempel, Sandra. *The Strange Case of the Broad Street Pump: John Snow and the Mystery of Cholera*. Berkeley: University of California Press, 2007.

Hoff, Brent, and Charles Smith III. *Mapping Epidemics: A Historical Atlas of Disease*. New York: Franklin Watts, 2000.

Hopkins, Donald R. *The Greatest Killer: Smallpox in History*. Chicago: University of Chicago Press, 2002.

Johnson, Niall. *Britain and the 1918–19 Influenza Epidemic: A Dark Epilogue*. New York: Routledge, 2006.

Johnson, Steven. *Ghost Map: The Story of London's Deadliest Epidemic*. New York: Penguin Group, 2006.

Karlen, Arno. *Man and Microbes: Disease and Plagues in History and Modern Times*. New York: Putnam, 1995.

Levenson, Jacob. *The Secret Epidemic: The Story of AIDS and Black America*. New York: Pantheon Books, 2004.

McKenna, Maryn. *Beating Back the Devil: On the Front Lines with the Disease Detectives of the Epidemic Intelligence Service*. New York: Free Press, 2004.

Murphy, Jim. *An American Plague: The True and Terrifying Story of the Yellow Fever Epidemic of 1793.* New York: Clarion Books, 2003.

Oldstone, Michael B. A. *Viruses, Plagues, and History.* New York: Oxford University Press, 2000.

Orr, Tamra. *Avian Flu.* New York: Rosen, 2007.

Oshinsky, David M. *Polio: An American Story.* New York: Oxford University Press, 2005.

Peters, C. J., and Mark Olshaker. *Virus Hunter: Thirty Years of Battling Hot Viruses Around the World.* New York: Anchor Books, 1997.

Preston, Richard. *The Demon in the Freezer.* New York: Random House, 2002.

———. *The Hot Zone.* New York: Random House, 1994.

Rice, Geoffrey W. *Black November: The 1918 Influenza Pandemic in New Zealand.* Christchurch: Canterbury University Press, 2005.

Shilts, Randy. *And the Band Played On: Politics, People, and the AIDS Epidemic.* New York: St. Martin's Press, 1987.

Walters, Mark Jerome. *Six Modern Plagues and How We Are Causing Them.* Washington, D.C.: Island Press/Shearwater Books, 2003.

Watts, Sheldon J. *Epidemics and History: Disease, Power, and Imperialism.* New Haven: Yale University Press, 1997.

Web Sites

Readers seeking additional information about global epidemics may wish to refer to the following Web sites, all of which were operational as of this writing.

Centers for Disease Control and Prevention (CDC)
www.cdc.gov

Affiliated with the U.S. Department of Health and Human Services, this oranization is the leading American government agency for protecting the public health of U.S. citizens. In addition to disseminating information about diseases and public health issues to the citizenry and state and local health departments, the CDC works to prevent the spread of infectious diseases.

Infectious Diseases Society of America (IDSA)
www.idsociety.org

The IDSA is a medical association representing physicians, scientists, and other health-care professionals who specialize in infectious diseases. This Web site provides information on improving health, including advice on preventing the spread of infectious diseases, among other issues.

The Journal of the American Medical Association (JAMA)
jama.ama-assn.org

Founded in 1883, *JAMA* is an international peer-reviewed medical journal, published 48 times a year by the American Medical Association. The most widely circulated medical journal in the country, it contains a wide variety of articles, including ones pertaining to epidemic outbreaks and infectious diseases.

National Institutes of Health (NIH)
www.nih.gov

Affiliated with the U.S. Department of Health and Human Services, the NIH is the primary agency of the U.S. government responsible for biomedical research.

The World Health Organization (WHO)
www.who.int/csr/en

On this Web site, a reader will find an Epidemic and Pandemic Alert and Response Guide provided by the WHO, an international public health authority working under the auspices of the United Nations and located in Geneva, Switzerland.

Additional Periodical Articles with Abstracts

More information about global epidemics and pandemics can be found in the following articles. Readers who are interested in additional articles may consult the *Readers' Guide to Periodical Literature* and other H.W. Wilson indexes and publications.

My Mother's Body. Mary Gordon. *The American Scholar,* v. 75 p63–78 Autumn 2006.

The writer considers the challenge of writing about her mother's body, which was afflicted with polio from a young age but retained many attractive features. She describes the eventual deterioration of her mother's body and her own difficulty in dealing with the process of her mother's disease. She also describes the way in which the scent of her mother's perfume generates memories of her mother and summons her presence.

Exquisite Plague. Aaron E. Hirsh. *The American Scholar*, v. 73 p113–17 Summer 2004.

The microbe Mycobacterium tuberculosis travels in minute particles—the tiny nuclei that puff from a cough and explode from a sneeze, according to Hirsh. When they are inhaled, these droplet nuclei sometimes travel past the trachea and the bronchi and eventually settle in the lung's deep, tiny pouches of air, where the microbe begins a complex subversion of human defenses. In fact, the microbe's first move is to vanish directly into the very last place it would be expected to hide: the macrophage, a cell developed specifically for the detection and eradication of invaders. Once inside, the microbe secretes a set of compounds that appear to hijack the membrane that transports it.

Notes from the 2006 AAAS Annual Meeting. Yvonne Baskin. *BioScience*, v. 56 p368 April 2006.

The writer discusses research presented at the annual meeting of the American Association for the Advancement of Science, held from February 16 to 20 in St. Louis, Missouri. Geographer William Woods of the University of Kansas, archaeologist Eduardo Neves of the University of Sao Paulo in Brazil, and biogeochemist Johannes Lehmann of Cornell University presented findings from studies into ancient people's enrichment of soils in Amazonia. Mark Woolhouse of the University of Edinburgh in Scotland presented findings from research into emerging human pathogens, and Alan Barrett of the University of Texas Medical Branch discussed the activity of the West Nile virus in the United States, Canada, Mexico, and the Caribbean.

Catastrophe in the Wings? Timothy M. Beardsley, *BioScience* v. 56 p179 March 2006.

Authorities on avian influenza are almost unanimous in believing that a global pandemic of the H5N1 strain of that disease, thought to have a 50 percent fatality rate in humans, is possible, if not likely, writes Beardsley. Emerging facts leave scant room for complacency. As of mid-February 2006, avian H5N1 cases had been logged in over a dozen countries in Asia, Europe, and Africa;

human infections, nearly all seemingly acquired directly from poultry, had been found in Cambodia, China, Indonesia, Iraq, Thailand, Turkey, and Vietnam. The chief fear of virologists is that H5N1 could undergo genetic reassortment in an individual harboring both H5N1 and a variant more easily transmitted among humans. The resulting hybrid could therefore blend easy human-to-human infection and high mortality. The influenza virus is notorious for abrupt alterations that confound acquired immunity.

The Next Pandemic. *Canada and the World Backgrounder*, v. 70 p10 December 2004.

According to the author of this article, nature's preferred means of reducing the population is the pandemic. The really terrifying pandemics are those for which no defenses or cures are available. The writer discusses fears about the proliferation of SARS, West Nile virus, and avian influenza.

Will the Black Death Return? Wendy Orent. *Discover,* v. 22 p72–77 November 2001.

Plague still has the potential to cause devastation, warns Orent. There have been three major epidemics of plague: Justinian's plague, which broke out in A.D. 542 and killed 100 million people in a 50-year period, the medieval Black Death, which probably killed one-quarter of all Europeans, and the Third Pandemic in Asia early in the 20th century, which killed 10 million people. Although plague is usually a sluggish disease that can only be transmitted by a flea infected with the bacterium *Yersinia pestis*, the speed of its spread during these pandemics indicates that, at times, the disease can become transmitted from human to human. The possibility that plague becomes more virulent and transmissible as it cycles in humans has terrifying implications given the development of an antibiotic-resistant plague in the 1980s by Russian bioweapons scientists. Although there is no evidence that anyone in Russia is still studying weapons strains, even genetically unmodified plague bombs would make a formidable terrorist weapon.

Megadeath in Mexico. Bruce Stutz. *Discover*, v. 27 p44–51 February 2006.

Mexican epidemiologist Rodolfo Acuna-Soto believes that the decimation of the Aztec population in the 16th century was not solely due to smallpox brought by Spanish colonizers, Stutz reports. Acuna-Soto's studies of ancient documents found that outbreaks of *zahuatl*—the Aztec word for smallpox—occurred in 1520 and 1531 but that the epidemics of 1545 and 1576 seemed to be another disease, called *cocolitzli*, which had the hallmarks of a hemorrhagic fever. Such diseases do not readily pass between people, so the virus must have been native rather than a Spanish import. Acuna-Soto then found that each of the *cocolitzli* epidemics occurred in the wet periods that followed several years of drought. Evidence from tree rings revealed that central Mexico suffered severe drought in the 16th century, with wet interludes around 1545 and 1576. Acuna-Soto thinks that a dormant hemorrhagic fever virus was spread by rodent populations that bred quickly when the rains returned after the drought.

Managing a Bird Flu Pandemic. Del Stover. *The Education Digest*, v. 71 p22–24 May 2006.

In an article condensed from the March 14 issue of *School Board News*, Stover expresses concern regarding a possible avian flu pandemic that could kill thousands or even millions. As the avian flu virus has spread around the world, health officials state that there is no immediate danger but note that an influenza pandemic takes place every 30 to 40 years, and prudence calls for planning now. That planning will more and more involve local school officials, who must get ready for the possibility of a major disruption in school operations. In a worst-case scenario, a pandemic could compel school closures and the transformation of school gyms and cafeterias into makeshift hospitals and make it necessary to find alternative ways to educate homebound children for a space of weeks or even months. The writer discusses the pandemic planning taking place among a number of schools.

Medical Countermeasures. *FDA Consumer*, v. 38 p24–27 January/February 2004.

The FDA is working to protect the U.S. against bioterrorism, according to the author of this article. To ensure that safe and effective products are available for diagnosing, treating, and preventing illness caused by terrorist agents, the FDA works with other agencies and manufacturers to identify promising research and encourage the development of new products. The agency also supports clinical research aimed at discovering whether products approved for one indication could be used for an indication related to counterterrorism, conducts its own research, and publishes guidelines for using medical countermeasures in specific groups. In certain circumstances, the FDA can also approve medical treatments against terrorist agents based on effectiveness data from animal studies alone. Countermeasures that are in place against a range of agents deemed to present the greatest threats to public health are discussed.

The Deadliest Virus. *Foreign Policy*, p20 January/February 2006.

In an interview, John Barry, author of *The Great Influenza: The Epic Story of the Deadliest Plague in History,* discusses President Bush's avian flu plan, measures to assist less-developed countries in combating the disease, the effect of a pandemic on trade and economic development, and the lessons to be learned from the government's inadequate response to Hurricane Katrina.

Remember SARS? This May Be Worse. Dan Hawaleshka. *Maclean's,* v. 119 p44–48 August 14–21, 2006.

Hawaleshka suggests that there may be hundreds of strains of the bacterium *Clostridium difficile (C. diff.)*, a superbug dubbed the epidemic strain. This hypervirulent variety has killed thousands of individuals, frequently elderly patients in hospitals, across North America over approximately the last five years, especially in Quebec, where it killed an estimated 2,000 patients in 2003–04 alone. Usually, the victims have been on antibiotics, which as well as fighting infection also kill the good bacteria normally found in the gastrointestinal tract. In their absence, *C. diff.* has no competition and flourishes. The link to recent exposure to antibiotics is so emphatic it is deemed a virtual pre-requisite for coming down with *C. diff.* Now, however, officials from the Centers for Disease Control and Prevention are worried by evidence indicating that *C. diff.* is spreading out of U.S. hospitals and into the community in general. The writer discusses the spread of the epidemic strain of *C. diff.*

In Oil-Rich Angola, Cholera Preys upon Poorest. Sharon LaFraniere. *New York Times*, pA1+ June 16, 2006.

Water supplies contaminated by raw sewage and garbage have caused cholera epidemics in Angola, reports LaFraniere. It is estimated that it has sickened 43,000 and killed 1,600 since February. Observers commented that the Angolan government is still unable to provide basic sanitation, even though it made a $2 billion surplus last year by selling crude oil.

U.S. Urges H.I.V. Tests for Adults and Teenagers. Donald McNeil. *New York Times*, pA1+ September 22, 2006.

McNeil reports that the federal government wants all teenagers and most adults to have H.I.V. tests as part of routine medical care, since many Americans who are infected with the AIDS virus don't know it. This is a shift in policy from the early days of the AIDS epidemic, when the stigma of the disease and the fear of social ostracism made many people avoid being tested.

The End of the World. John Acocella. *The New Yorker*, v. 81 p82–85 March 21, 2005.

Acocella reviews *The Great Mortality: An Intimate History of the Black Death, the Most Devastating Plague of All Time*, by science writer John Kelly, and *In the Wake of the Plague: The Black Death and the World It Made*, by Norman Cantor. Kelly's book is one of the latest titles to deal with the pandemic of bubonic plague that hit Europe in the mid-14th century. It contains much interesting information, but there is a weakness in his narrative plan, which generally involves going region by region, city by city. There is little information for some municipalities and a sameness of information for others, with the result that Kelly is forced to pad and sometimes to fictionalize. In *In the Wake of the Plague*, Cantor is at his best when writing about human psychology, particularly as its medieval contours differed from ours. The weakest part of Cantor's book is his summary of the various theories of the Black Death that have accumulated over the years.

Bracing for a Plague. Geoffrey Cowley. *Newsweek*, v. 146 p72+ December 12, 2005.

In an interview with Cowley, David Nabarro, the UN's senior coordinator for avian and human influenza, discusses the challenges of his job, the development of a simulation network to examine possible progressions of a flu outbreak, the lessons that have been learned from previous epidemics, whether countries that lack functioning health systems can afford to invest for potential health problems, his opinion of the Bush administration's new $7 billion preparedness plan, and whether he enjoys his work.

The New World of Global Health. Jon Cohen. *Science*, v. 311 p162–67 January 13, 2006.

Cohen writes that the limitations of recent ambitious efforts to tackle infectious diseases of the poor are becoming apparent. Over the last seven years, a group of rich, impassioned players, such as the Bill and Melinda Gates Foundation, have committed over $35 billion to fighting the diseases of the world's poor. However, such organizations are now going through a period of increased external scrutiny and internal soul-searching over what they are actually achieving. The objectives of these organizations are hugely, even impossibly, ambitious, and accomplishing these objectives is proving tougher than many expected because of such factors as bureaucracy, corruption, and a lack of trained health-care workers. In addition, these organizations are struggling with issues of accountability, credit, and even fundamental direction, and considerable confusion exists over how they should mesh with each other and with older agencies.

What Links Bats to Emerging Infectious Diseases? Andrew P. Dobson. *Science*, v. 310 p628–29 October 28, 2005.

Knowing more about bat ecology and immunology is crucial to determining the threat imposed by new pathogens, according to Dobson. Three species of horseshoe bats (*Rhinolophus spp.*) have now been officially recorded as the natural reservoir host of the coronavirus that causes severe acute respiratory syndrome (SARS). Moreover, bats are now known to be natural reservoir hosts to various other disease pathogens, both established and emergent. Pathogens that use bats as reservoirs are likely transmitted to new hosts through infected fruit remnants that bats spit out. It is essential to recognize that increased rates of spillover-mediated pathogen transmission from bats to humans may result from increased bat-human contact through anthropogenic modification of the bat's natural environment.

Genome Sequence Diversity and Clues to the Evolution of Variola (Smallpox) Virus. Joseph J. Esposito, Scott A. Sammons, and A. Michael Frace. *Science,* v. 313 p807–12 August 11, 2006.

The authors note that comparative genomics of 45 epidemiologically varied variola virus isolates from the last 30 years of the smallpox era indicate low sequence diversity, suggesting that there is probably little difference in the isolates' functional gene content. Phylogenetic clustering inferred three clades coincident with their geographical origin and case-fatality rate; the latter implicated putative proteins that mediate viral virulence differences. Analysis of the viral linear DNA genome suggests that its evolution involved direct descent and DNA end-region recombination events. Knowing the sequences will help scientists understand the viral proteome and improve diagnostic test precision, therapeutics, and systems for their assessment.

Target Practice. Aimee Cunningham. *Science News*, v. 170 p152–53 September 2, 2006.

According to Cunningham, researchers are trying to develop new treatments to fight tuberculosis. One-third of the world's population is infected with

Mycobacterium tuberculosis, which kills more people than any other single infectious bacterium, and the incidence of multidrug-resistant tuberculosis is steadily increasing. Several groups are focusing on the bacterium's cell wall, which is packed with extra layers of sugars and lipids, making it almost impenetrable to the human immune system and many antibiotics. Others are targeting genes that coordinate the bacterium's internal resistance and the metabolic pathways that keep it alive day to day. Many biochemical and technical challenges remain to be overcome on the path to better treatments, but increased funding in recent years means that many scientists are confident that progress can be achieved.

Model Explains Bubonic Plague's Persistence. John Travis. *Science News*, v. 158 p262 October 21, 2000.

In the October 19, 2000, issue of *Nature*, Travis writes, Keeling and Gilligan come to the counterintuitive conclusion that killing rats may intensify bubonic plague outbreaks among people. Keeling and Gilligan's computer model mirrors historical records of plague epidemics in medieval Europe by showing human outbreaks about every decade. The model suggests that the best way for prevention of the bubonic plague in people is to stop its spread in rats and that killing rats once the disease has spread to humans will release many infected fleas. The researchers hope to extend the model to establish the circumstances under which the disease could spread to rats in U.S. cities.

An Uncertain Defense. W. Wayt Gibbs. *Scientific American*, v. 291 p20+ October 2004.

Many new antibioweapons vaccines, such as a new Ebola vaccine, will not be tested in humans, reports Gibbs. On July 21, 2004, President Bush signed the Project BioShield Act, which authorizes the Department of Homeland Security to spend as much as $5.6 billion over 10 years to increase its stockpile of antibioweapons medications and which specifically mandates the stockpiling of an untested Ebola vaccine. Not having undergone human clinical trials, many of these drugs have not yet been approved as safe or effective by the FDA, and the treatment of thousands of people with medications that have undergone only animal studies may be risky.

A Strategy of Containment. Christine Soares. *Scientific American*, v. 290 p48+ March 2004.

Soares profiles David L. Heymann, head of the WHO's polio eradication program. Heymann was recruited into the WHO's smallpox eradication program after leaving the London School of Hygiene and Tropical Medicine in 1974. In 1976 he joined the CDC's epidemic intelligence service, where he became involved in the first case of Legionnaire's disease and was sent to Zaire to investigate an Ebola virus outbreak. In 1995 Heymann was charged with creating an emerging and infectious disease program by the WHO, and he became head of the polio program in July 2003.

Planning for the Pandemic. Stefanie Friedhoff. *Time*, v. 167 p57 March 20, 2006.

The writer looks at the epidemiologist Sandro Galea, who studies human minds and how they might respond to an outbreak of a disease such as SARS, Ebola, or avian flu. Galea is one of the pioneers of the public psychology of emerging diseases, a new field of research. As professor of epidemiology at the University of Michigan's School of Public Health, Galea has studied the way in which Canadians responded to the 2003 SARS outbreak and quarantines in Toronto.

An African Miracle. Christine Gorman. *Time*, v. 168 p96–98 December 4, 2006.

Gorman explains that a few doctors have used antiretroviral (ARV) drugs to turn around the lives of thousands of children with AIDS. For years, administering ARVs to children suffering from AIDS in the least developed regions of the world was considered a lost cause, but now thousands of African children are receiving the lifesaving treatment they need. Researchers revealed that children react faster and better than adults to ARVs. Groups such as President Bush's Emergency Plan for AIDS Relief, the Clinton Foundation, and a few nonprofit organizations, corporations, and faith-based groups have risen to the challenge. The writer discusses the case of Bokang Rakabaele, an eight-year-old South African boy suffering from AIDS, tuberculosis, and pneumonia whose health has improved dramatically in the past six months due to his treatment with ARVs.

The Bird Flu: Are We Ready for a Pandemic? Jane Lloyd. *UN Chronicle*, v. 42 p64+ December 2005/February 2006.

Lloyd reports that David Heymann, assistant director-general of the World Health Organization, claims that the threat of a pandemic influenza extends to all known countries. Heymann was one of a group of international experts who convened at UN Headquarters in New York to discuss the threat the disease poses for people worldwide, along with strategies to tackle the virus, with an emphasis on UN involvement. He reports that, because the virus is new to humans and causes illness or death, it has only to establish the capacity to spread easily from human to human to fulfill the three criteria required for a pandemic to start. According to Louise Fresco, assistant director-general of the Food and Agricultural Organization (FAO) of the UN, the FAO believes that eliminating avian influenza among poultry can postpone or stop the development of the H5N1 virus into a form capable of creating a human pandemic. The writer discusses the threat posed by avian flu and the measures proposed to combat it.

The AIDS Crisis: Address to XVI International AIDS Conference. Bill Clinton. *Vital Speeches of the Day*, v. 72 p716–21 November 2006.

Former U.S. president Bill Clinton, in addressing the XVI International AIDS Conference in Toronto, Canada, claimed that much has been achieved in the global fight against HIV/AIDS, but much remains to be done. Four years ago, he said, there were 6 million people in developing nations in desperate need of livesaving treatment, and outside Brazil, fewer than 70,000 were getting the necessary medication. Today, over 1.3 million are receiving treatment, but that figure will soon reach 3 million and beyond, and many nations experienced a decline in infection among young people in 2005. Nonetheless, more money needs to be spent more effectively, Clinton said. He maintained that prevention efforts have to be stepped up, more voluntary testing needs to be conducted, women's status must be lifted, the search for medical answers through microbiocides and vaccines must be continued, difficult-to-reach populations must be reached, and the infrastructure required to get treatment to everyone who needs it has to be developed.

Index